QUIK-CARD for Blood Gas Interpretation

Normal arterial range, sea level, FIO_2, 0.21

pH	7.35–7.45
$PaCO_2$	35–45 mm Hg
PaO_2	70–100 mm Hg (age-depend.)
SaO_2	93–98%
HCO_3^-	22–26 mEq/L
% MetHb	< 2.0%
% COHb	< 3.0%
Base excess	−2.0 to 2.0 mEq/L
CaO_2	16–22 mL O_2/dL

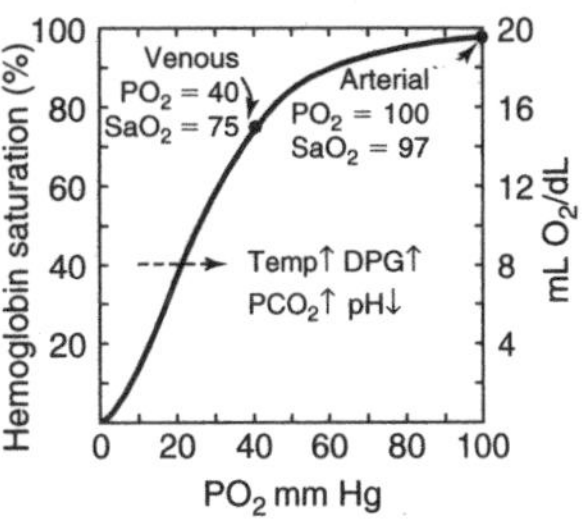

Eq. 1) $PaCO_2 = \dfrac{\dot{V}CO_2 \times 0.863}{\dot{V}A}$

$\dot{V}CO_2$ = CO_2 prod./min; $\dot{V}A = \dot{V}E - \dot{V}D = f(V_T - V_D)$. f = resp. rate, V_T and V_D = tidal & dead space volume.

↑ $PaCO_2$ can arise from:

Inadequate $\dot{V}E$ (↓f &/or ↓$\dot{V}_T$)	Increased $\dot{V}D$
CNS drugs	Parenchymal lung disease (V-Q imbal.)
Respiratory muscle weakness	Rapid, shallow breathing
Central hypoventilation	

$PaCO_2$	Condition in blood	State of alveolar ventilation
> 45 mm Hg	Hypercapnia	Hypoventilation
35–45 mm Hg	Eucapnia	Normal ventilation
< 35 mm Hg	Hypocapnia	Hyperventilation

NOTES: (1) There is no predictable correlation between $PaCO_2$ and resp. rate, V_T, or clinical appearance, since they do not indicate either CO_2 production or alveolar ventilation. (2) ↑ $PaCO_2$ ⟶ ↓ PAO_2 (see Eq. 2, alveolar gas eq.) and ↓ PaO_2. (3) ↑ $PaCO_2$ ⟶ ↓ pH (see Eq. 4, H-H eq.)

Eq. 2) Alveolar PO_2 (PAO_2) = FIO_2 (P_B − 47) − 1.2($PaCO_2$)

Alveolar-arterial PO_2 difference (A-a Gradient) = PAO_2 − PaO_2 = $P(A\text{-}a)O_2$

NOTES: (1) PaO_2 varies with PAO_2, so you cannot properly interpret any PaO_2 without knowledge of PAO_2 variables: P_B, FIO_2, and $PaCO_2$. (2) Normal $P(A\text{-}a)O_2$ ↑ with ↑ FIO_2 and ↑ age. Abnormal $P(A\text{-}a)O_2$ = lung disorder or anatomic shunt. (3) Normal $P(A\text{-}a)O_2$: On room air = (3 + 0.21 × age in yrs.) ± 5 mm Hg
On FIO_2 of 1.00, upper limit of normal is 120 mm Hg

Eq. 3) CaO_2 (O_2 content) = O_2 bound to Hb + O_2 dissolved in plasma
(mL O_2/dL) = (Hb × 1.34 × SaO_2) + (0.003 × PaO_2)

CAUSES OF HYPOXEMIA (low PaO_2, SaO_2, or CaO_2)[1]

Respiratory	PaO_2	$P(A\text{-}a)O_2$	SaO_2[2]	CaO_2
Pulmonary right to left shunt	Decr	Incr	Decr	Decr
Ventilation-perfusion (V-Q) imbalance	Decr	Incr	Decr	Decr
Diffusion barrier [3]	Decr	Incr	Decr	Decr
Hypoventilation (↑ $PaCO_2$)	Decr	Nl	Decr	Decr
Nonrespiratory				
Cardiac right-to-left shunt	Decr	Incr	Decr	Decr
Decreased PIO_2[4]	Decr	Nl	Decr	Decr
Low mixed venous O_2 content (CvO_2) [5]	Nl	Nl	Nl	Nl
Anemia [6]	Nl	Nl	Decr	Decr
Carbon monoxide excess [7]	Nl	Nl	Decr	Decr
Methemoglobin excess [7]	Nl	Nl	Decr	Decr

NOTES: (1) Nl = normal; Decr = decreased; Incr = increased. (2) SaO_2 relates to PaO_2 by O_2 diss. curve (see graph, top; CaO_2 shown for Hb =15 g/dL%). Curve shifts to R with ↓ pH, ↑ PCO_2, ↑ 2,3 DPG, & ↑ temp.; opposites shift curve to L. (3) Changes shown clinically important only with ↑ pulmonary blood flow (e.g., exercise). (4) ↓ PIO_2 from ↓ barometric press. or ↓ FIO_2. (5) Low CvO_2 can reduce PaO_2, SaO_2, and CaO_2 if there is increased venous admixture. (6) Reduced Hb does not affect PaO_2 or SaO_2, unless there is increased venous admixture, but will lower CaO_2 (see Eq. 3). (7) Excess COHb & MetHb will ↓ SaO_2 but not PaO_2; SaO_2 may appear falsely normal if calculated from PaO_2 or measured by pulse oximetry; must measure SaO_2 by co-oximetry on blood sample.

Eq. 4) Henderson-Hasselbalch Equation

$$pH = pK + \log \frac{[HCO_3^-]}{0.03\,[PaCO_2]}$$

Acidemia: blood pH < 7.35
Acidosis: a primary physiologic process that tends to cause acidemia.
Alkalemia: blood pH > 7.45
Alkalosis: a primary physiologic process that tends to cause alkalemia.

FOUR PRIMARY ACID-BASE DISORDERS (a-b dis.): DEFINITIONS, SOME CLINICAL CAUSES, AND EXPECTED DEGREE OF COMPENSATION

First Change | Compensation

$\downarrow pH \cong \frac{*HCO_3^-}{\uparrow PaCO_2}$ $\quad \uparrow pH \cong \frac{\uparrow HCO_3^-}{\uparrow PaCO_2}$

Respiratory acidosis—A primary a-b dis. in which the 1st change is an elevation of $PaCO_2$, resulting in decreased pH; compensation is renal retention of bicarbonate.

SOME CAUSES OF RESP. ACIDOSIS: Central nervous system depression (e.g., drug overdose), chest bellows dysfunction (e.g., myasthenia gravis), disease of lungs and/or airways (e.g., asthma, COPD, pulmonary edema).

COMPENSATION FOR RESP. ACIDOSIS: For each 10 mm Hg ↑ in $PaCO_2$:
*Acute ⟶ HCO_3^- ↑ by ~ 1 mEq/L (due to biochemical buffering), pH ↓ by ~ 0.07.
Compensated (days) ⟶ HCO_3^- ↑ by 3-4 mEq/L, pH ↓ by ~ 0.03.

$\uparrow pH \cong \frac{**HCO_3^-}{\downarrow PaCO_2}$ $\quad \uparrow pH \cong \frac{\downarrow HCO_3^-}{\downarrow PaCO_2}$

Respiratory alkalosis—A primary a-b dis. in which the 1st change is a lowering of $PaCO_2$, resulting in elevated pH; compensation is renal excretion of bicarbonate.

SOME CAUSES OF RESP. ALKALOSIS: Hypoxemia (includes altitude), pulmonary embolism, anxiety, sepsis, liver failure, any acute pulmonary condition.

COMPENSATION FOR RESP. ALKALOSIS: For each 10 mm Hg ↓ in $PaCO_2$:
**Acute ⟶ HCO_3^- ↓ by ~ 2 mEq/L (due to biochemical buffering), pH ↑ by ~ 0.08.
Compensated (days) ⟶ HCO_3^- ↓ by ~ 5 mEq/L, pH ↑ by ~ 0.03.

$\downarrow pH \cong \frac{\downarrow HCO_3^-}{PaCO_2}$ $\quad \uparrow pH \cong \frac{\downarrow HCO_3^-}{\downarrow PaCO_2}$

Metabolic acidosis—A primary a-b dis. in which the 1st change is a lowering of HCO_3^-, resulting in decreased pH; compensation is hyperventilation.

SOME CAUSES OF MET. ACIDOSIS: With ↑ anion gap: lactic acidosis, ketoacidosis, some poisons (ethylene glycol, methanol), some overdoses (aspirin, isoniazid). With normal anion gap: diarrhea, interstitial nephritis, renal tubular acidosis.

COMPENSATION FOR MET. ACIDOSIS: When fully compensated (> 12 hrs.): Expected $PaCO_2$ = (1.5 × serum CO_2) + (8 ± 2); *or* last two digits of pH = $PaCO_2$ ± 2 (e.g., pH 7.25, $PaCO_2$ 25 ± 2).

$\uparrow pH \cong \frac{\uparrow HCO_3^-}{PaCO_2}$ $\quad \uparrow pH \cong \frac{\uparrow HCO_3^-}{\uparrow PaCO_2}$

Metabolic alkalosis—A primary a-b dis. in which the 1st change is elevation of HCO_3^-, resulting in increased pH; compensation is hypoventilation.

SOME CAUSES OF MET. ALKALOSIS: Chloride-therapy responsive: contraction alkalosis, diuretics, corticosteroids, gastric suctioning, vomiting. Chloride-therapy resistant: any hyperaldosterone state, e.g., Cushing syndrome, Bartter syndrome, severe K^+ depletion.

COMPENSATION FOR MET. ALKALOSIS: Least predictable compensation of the four primary disorders; for every mEq/L increase in HCO_3^-, there may be 0.6–0.7 mm Hg increase in $PaCO_2$.

DIAGNOSING MIXED ACID-BASE DISORDERS

1. Examine serum electrolytes (Na^+, K^+, Cl^-, CO_2). Calculate anion gap (AG), Δ AG, Δ CO_2, and the bicarbonate gap.
   AG = Na^+ − (Cl^- + CO_2); normal 12 ± 4 mEq/L (may vary with lab)
   Δ AG = AG − 12
   Δ CO_2 = 27 − venous CO_2
   Bicarbonate gap = Δ AG − Δ CO_2 = Na^+ − Cl^- − 39 (normal 0 ± 6 mEq/L)
   > + 6 = metabolic alkalosis &/or HCO_3^- retention for resp. acidosis
   < − 6 = hyperchloremic metabolic acidosis &/or HCO_3^- excretion for resp. alkalosis
2. Examine arterial blood gases. Single acid-base disorders do not compensate to normal blood pH. Normal pH with abnormal $PaCO_2$ &/or HCO_3^- = two or more primary disorders. If pH abnormal, determine if other values fit a single disorder or suggest a mixed disorder (see expected compensation, above).
3. Use a full clinical assessment (history, physical exam, other lab data) to explain the apparent acid-base disorder(s) in terms of clinical causes (see causes, above).
4. Treat the underlying clinical cause(s).
5. Aim toward correcting pH, especially if < 7.30, > 7.52 ([H^+] > 50, < 30 nM/L).

CLINICAL JUDGMENT SHOULD ALWAYS APPLY

SECOND EDITION

All You Really Need to Know to Interpret Arterial Blood Gases

SECOND EDITION

All You Really Need to Know to Interpret Arterial Blood Gases

Lawrence Martin, M.D., FACP, FCCP
Chief, Division of Pulmonary and Critical Care Medicine
Mt. Sinai Medical Center, Cleveland
Associate Professor of Medicine
Case Western Reserve University School of Medicine

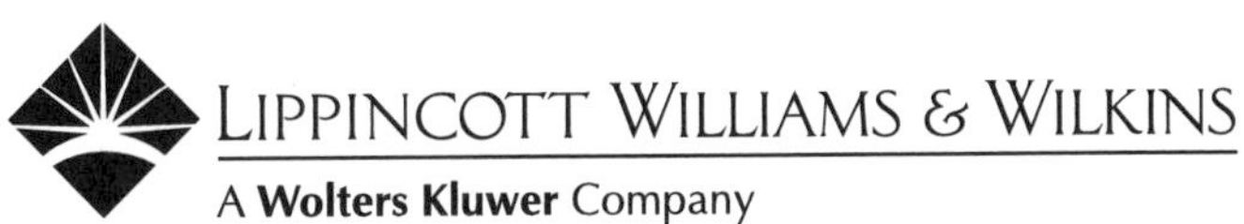

Philadelphia • Baltimore • New York • London
Buenos Aires • Hong Kong • Sydney • Tokyo

Editor: Craig Percy
Managing Editor: Tanya Lazar
Marketing Manager: Melissa Harris
Project Editor: Kathleen Gilbert

351 West Camden Street
Baltimore, Maryland 21201-2436 USA

227 East Washington Square
Philadelphia, PA 19106

The publisher is not responsible (as a matter of product liability, negligence or otherwise) for any injury resulting from any material contained herein. This publication contains information relating to general principles of medical care which should not be construed as specific instructions for individual patients. Manufacturers' product information and package inserts should be reviewed for current information, including contraindications, dosages and precautions.

Printed in Canada

First Edition, 1992

Library of Congress Cataloging-in-Publication Data

Martin, Lawrence, 1943-
All you really need to know to interpret arterial blood gases / edited by Lawrence Martin.
p. cm.
Includes bibliographical references and index.
ISBN 0–683–30604–9
1. Blood gases—Analysis
RB45. 2 .M37 1999
616.07'561—dc21

98–48608
CIP

The publishers have made every effort to trace the copyright holders for borrowed material. If they have inadvertently overlooked any, they will be pleased to make the necessary arrangements at the first opportunity.

To purchase additional copies of this book, call our customer service department at **(800) 638-3030** or fax orders to **(301) 824-7390.** International customers should call **(301) 714-2324.**

99 00 01 02
1 2 3 4 5 6 7 8 9 10

Disclaimer

This book is about how to interpret arterial blood gas data in the clinical setting. Although many patient examples are included, no book, including this one, can tell what to do in a specific clinical situation. Depending on the clinical setting, identical blood gas results can lead to very different clinical strategies. The author accepts no responsibility for any action or inaction on the part of any individual that may be based on information in this book.

To the medical students and house officers I have taught,
in appreciation for all they have taught me.

And to Joanna, my favorite medical student.

A Basic Test: Preface to the First Edition

There are a few basic tests used in the care of patients. A basic test is one that is applicable to a broad group of patients, provides invaluable information quickly, can be repeated as often as necessary, and is not dependent on patient effort for accuracy. My short list of such essential tests (in alphabetical order):

1. arterial blood gases
2. chest x-ray
3. complete blood count (CBC)
4. electrocardiogram
5. Gram's stain for bacteria
6. serum electrolytes, BUN and glucose
7. urine analysis.

No doubt, the better we understand information provided by these few tests, the better we can care for our patients. CT scans, echocardiograms, perfusion scans, Doppler studies, enzyme assays, spirometry, and other tests of specific organ function (e.g., thyroid, liver, pancreas) certainly have their place, and are at times crucial to diagnosis. However the seven tests listed above, along with the medical history and physical examination, form a foundation for managing virtually all inpatients and a great many chronically ill outpatients.

The newest test on this list to become routinely available is arterial blood gases. The first arterial puncture was performed in 1912 by Hurter, a German physician. In 1919 arterial blood gas analysis was first used as a diagnostic procedure. Employing Hurter's radial artery puncture technique, W.C. Stadie measured oxygen saturation in patients with pneumonia and showed that cyanosis of critically ill patients resulted from incomplete oxygenation of hemoglobin (Stadie 1919).

Over the next 40 years blood gas measurements were more of a laboratory research tool than a test available for everyday patient care. Techniques for measuring blood gases required specialized apparatus and were difficult to perform. It was not until the 1950s that electrodes were developed that could rapidly and reproducibly measure PaO_2, $PaCO_2$ and pH.

In 1953 Leland Clark invented the platinum oxygen electrode, a prototype that evolved into the first modern blood gas electrode (Clark 1953, Clark 1956). Development of commercially viable pH and PCO_2 electrodes soon followed and by the mid-1960s several university centers were able to provide pH, $PaCO_2$ and PaO_2 measurements on arterial blood, albeit using cumbersome and non-automated equipment. In 1973 the first commercially available, automated blood gas machine was introduced (ABL1 from Radiometer), and this was soon followed by machines from other companies (Severinghaus 1986). Today virtually every acute care hospital provides rapid and automated blood gas testing 24 hours a day, 7 days a week.

As performed by electrodes on a single sample of arterial blood, the ABG test now has competition: non-invasive measurements. Particularly popular, and replacing the need for some arterial sample-based tests, are pulse oximeters for measuring oxygen saturation and end-tidal gas analysis for PCO_2. In neonates and small children, skin electrodes for measuring PO_2 and PCO_2 have found wide application. Even more exciting is the new technology for measuring blood gases *continuously,* using tiny fiberoptic sensors that fit inside the blood vessel. Although an invasive technique, optical sensing promises to add a new dimension to monitoring changes in pH, $PaCO_2$ and PaO_2.

Whatever the technology, the important thing is the information and its proper clinical application. All blood gas technologies are designed to provide information on oxygenation, ventilation and/or acid–base balance through one or more measurements. Teaching you how to interpret and wisely use blood gas values—no matter how they are obtained—is the goal of this book.

This is not a physiology textbook. I have left out some aspects of blood gas physiology that, while interesting, are not crucial to learning basic blood gas interpretation; examples include the shunt equation, the carbon dioxide dissociation curve, and the Fick equation for oxygen uptake. Nor is this a compendium of all clinical situations. Omitted are discussions of blood gases during the neonatal period, mixed venous oxygen measurements, and blood gas alterations during hyperbaric therapy. The bibliography provides several references where one can find discussion of these and other specialized topics.

Rather than produce an encyclopedia that covers everything lightly, I have tried to create a work that will, first and foremost, teach the important aspects in depth and be clinically useful. The vast majority of people who use arterial blood gases in the care of patients should find in this book all they "really need to know."

Lawrence Martin, M.D.
Cleveland

Preface to the Second Edition

In the field of blood gas interpretation, not much has changed since the first edition of this book (in 1992). The basic physiology is the same, of course, and the way the test is run is also little changed. A new edition is nonetheless justified for several reasons.

First, there is the need to incorporate additional information on noninvasive "blood gas" data, principally pulse oximetry measurement of SpO_2 and end-tidal PCO_2 ($PetCO_2$) monitoring. Both tests have now become routine in the management of patients, the $PetCO_2$ mainly in the intensive care arena. These tests are largely responsible for a nationwide decline in the number of arterial samples analyzed for blood gas data. Indeed, it is now commonplace to manage stable, mechanically ventilated patients almost entirely without arterial blood draws, using only noninvasive blood gas measurements. Expanded coverage of this topic is included within the respective chapters on PCO_2 and oxygen saturation.

A new edition also provides me with the opportunity to better explain some important physiology. For example, in discussions with students and physicians, I often encounter confusion about the crucial differences between PaO_2, SaO_2, and oxygen content. The confusion is over how they relate to each other and to factors such as anemia, carboxyhemoglobin, and methemoglobin. This subject has been rewritten and greatly expanded for clarity and emphasis. Likewise, the section on anion gap and electrolytes has been expanded; several examples are provided on use of the bicarbonate gap to uncover mixed acid–base disorders.

I have also added a third "Putting It Altogether" chapter; this one is on clinical evaluation and test ordering. The two "Putting It Altogether" chapters in the first edition gave blood gas data to interpret, but did not ask when a blood gas is necessary and whether some other test could substitute. The new chapter presents 16 brief patient scenarios, most *without* any blood gas data, and you are asked to determine what gas exchange tests should be obtained: e.g., complete arterial blood gas measurements, co-oximetry alone, pulse oximetry alone, or no tests at all.

In the first edition, I omitted discussion of venous blood gases because, in my opinion, this is not information most clinicians really need to know. Yet many students and clinicians want to learn about this topic, even though they are seldom called on to interpret mixed venous blood gases. For them I have added the chapter "Venous Blood Gases: Beyond All You Really Need to Know."

Other changes to this edition include more figures, expansion of the pre-tests and post-tests, an enlarged reference section, and an Internet address for our pulmonary medicine World Wide Web site.

As always, emphasis is on basic gas exchange physiology useful in the care of patients. You will need a pencil to get the most out of this book, but a calculator is not necessary (though it may speed up problem solving). If you do the exercises as they are presented, you cannot help but learn "All You Really Need to Know to Interpret Arterial Blood Gases." I will go one step further: If you read carefully through each chapter and work on all the problems and exercises, you should acquire sufficient expertise to *teach* the subject.

Lawrence Martin, M.D., FACP, FCCP
Cleveland
martin@lightstream.net

The Internet

Since publication of the first edition I, like many others, have learned about the Internet and the World Wide Web and have embraced them as potentially valuable teaching tools. Our Mt. Sinai Hospital Pulmonary Division has developed an educational Web site covering a wide range of topics, including blood gas interpretation, the basics of pulmonary physiology, and the history of oxygen therapy. The site also contains my clickable e-mail address (martin@lightstream.net) in several places. The Web address is

http://www.mtsinai.org/pulmonary

Contents

How to Use This Book for Maximum Benefit

- Get a pencil.

  This is a very practical book about an important laboratory test: arterial blood gases. The book's emphasis is on interpreting blood gases in the clinical setting. Real patients and real clinical situations are presented along the way.

  Don't read this book without a pencil in hand. You will short change yourself if you do. You won't need a calculator, and blank paper is optional; the necessary arithmetic can be done in the book itself. *But go get a pencil.* Without applying pencil to paper—to answer the Clinical Problems and other questions before checking your answers—you won't be forced to think about the information presented. And you won't get the maximum value out of the book.

  In most of the chapters, you will encounter numbered Clinical Problems, each in a box; answers to these problems are at the end of their chapter. Additional questions for you to answer in the text are heralded by a ❓ ; these are answered in the paragraphs immediately following the question.

  Problems and questions:
  Numbered Clinical Problems: answered at the end of the chapter
  Not numbered (❓): answered in following paragraphs

  I recommend that you answer *all* the problems and questions with a pencil as they are encountered, then check your answers. Follow this advice and you cannot help but learn the fundamentals of blood gas interpretation. If you skip the pencil you won't know whether the information has registered or if you have really learned what's important. Applying pencil to paper is the only reliable way to *learn* what the book can teach you.

  So go get a pencil.
- Take the Pre-Test, then check your answers in Appendix B.
- Read "Introduction to ABG Quik-Course" on page xxiii. Then either review the Quik-Course or begin the book with Chapter 1.

- Read the chapters at your own pace, always stopping to answer each question *using your pencil.*
- Make sure you understand all the questions and answers in a given chapter before proceeding to the next chapter.
- Check the list of symbols or the glossary for any unfamiliar terms (Appendices C and D).
- Take the Post-Test after completing all the chapters (Appendix A).
- Write or e-mail me with any corrections, disagreements, suggestions for improvements, etc.

Lawrence Martin, M.D.
Chief, Division of Pulmonary and
Critical Care Medicine
Mt. Sinai Medical Center
One Mt. Sinai Drive
Cleveland, Ohio 44106
Fax: 216–421-6952
e-mail: martin@lightstream.net

Blood Gas Pre-Test

Take this test now. If you answer 90% or better of the 100 items correctly, give this book to a friend. You probably don't need it.

Directions: For each of the following 10 numbered statements or questions, **there may be none, one, or more than one correct response.** Circle the correct letter response(s) *before* checking the answers in Appendix B.

1. The normal range for $PaCO_2$ is 35–45 mm Hg. A sudden change in $PaCO_2$ from normal to 28 mm Hg means the subject
   a. Is hyperventilating
   b. Has excess alveolar ventilation for the amount of CO_2 production
   c. Must be breathing faster than normal
   d. Must have acute respiratory alkalosis
   e. Has reached a new steady state for gas exchange
2. Which of the following statements about $PaCO_2$ (arterial PCO_2) is(are) true?
   a. $PaCO_2$ is directly related to the rate of CO_2 production and inversely related to alveolar ventilation
   b. If $PaCO_2$ goes up, while the inspired air remains unchanged as to pressure and oxygen percentage, PaO_2 will go down
   c. Even when $PaCO_2 > 120$ mm Hg, it is possible to maintain a normal arterial oxygen saturation with inhaled supplemental oxygen
   d. In patients with lung disease, useful bedside parameters for determining whether $PaCO_2$ is high or low are respiratory rate and mental status exam
   e. To reach the summit of Mount Everest (barometric pressure 253 mm Hg) without supplemental oxygen and survive, one must keep the $PaCO_2 < 20$ mm Hg
3. The arterial PO_2 is predicted to be reduced to some extent from
   a. Anemia

b. Ventilation–perfusion (V–Q) imbalance with an increase in the number of low V–Q units
c. Increased $PaCO_2$, while the subject is breathing room air
d. Carbon monoxide poisoning
e. Increasing altitude

4. Which of the following sets of values would be helpful in assessing the acid–base state of a patient's blood?
   a. pH and $PaCO_2$
   b. pH and PaO_2
   c. $PaCO_2$ and PaO_2
   d. $PaCO_2$ and HCO_3^-
   e. pH and SaO_2

5. Which of the following statements regarding acid–base balance (is) are correct?
   a. HCO_3^- increases with acute elevation of $PaCO_2$, before any renal compensation takes place
   b. A patient can have metabolic acidosis and metabolic alkalosis at the same time
   c. A patient can have high anion gap metabolic acidosis and hyperchloremic metabolic acidosis at the same time
   d. An anion gap $\geq$ 20 mEq/L is presumptive evidence for metabolic acidosis unless proven otherwise
   e. In theory, the bicarbonate value calculated from the Henderson–Hasselbalch equation and the serum CO_2 value measured with serum electrolytes in venous blood should be identical

6. Which of the following statement(s) about PaO_2 (arterial PO_2) is(are) correct?
   a. In the absence of any right-to-left shunting of blood, PaO_2 is determined solely by the alveolar PO_2 and the interface of the alveoli and pulmonary capillaries
   b. PaO_2 is the sole determinant of SaO_2
   c. Oxygen molecules chemically bound to hemoglobin do not exert a gas pressure
   d. In a mountain climber with normal cardiopulmonary system, the decline in PaO_2 with increasing altitude is solely attributable to the fall in barometric pressure
   e. The PO_2 in a cup of water open to the atmosphere is always higher than the PaO_2 in a healthy person (breathing room air) who is holding the cup

7. Which of the following information, *including numerical values and units,* is(are) accurate and/or useful when determining a patient's arterial oxygen content (CaO_2)?
   a. Each 100 mL of hemoglobin can combine with 1.34 mL of oxygen
   b. Normal CaO_2 is between 16 and 22 mg/dL
   c. Normally, dissolved oxygen constitutes < 2.0% of the CaO_2
   d. Normally, mixed venous oxygen content at rest is about 25% less than CaO_2
   e. A 10% decrease in SaO_2 will produce the same percentage decrease in hemoglobin-bound oxygen content as will a 10% decrease in hemoglobin content

8. Arterial blood gas data (pH, $PaCO_2$, PaO_2, SaO_2) are related in some simple but important ways. Which of the following relationships is(are) valid?
   a. Alveolar PO_2 is related to $PaCO_2$ by the alveolar gas equation: as $PaCO_2$ goes up, alveolar PO_2 goes down
   b. PaO_2 is inversely related to blood pH: as pH goes up, PaO_2 goes down
   c. If $PaCO_2$ increases while HCO_3^- remains unchanged, pH always goes down
   d. PaO_2 is related to SaO_2 on a linear scale (i.e., a straight-line relationship)
   e. The SaO_2 is related to hemoglobin-bound arterial oxygen content on a linear scale (i.e., a straight-line relationship)

9. There are some truisms in terminology and physiology for proper blood gas interpretation. Which of the following statements is(are) true?
   a. *Hyperventilation* and *hypoventilation* are clinical terms and are not diagnosed by arterial blood gases
   b. The alveolar–arterial PO_2 difference increases with age and with increase in the fraction of inspired oxygen
   c. The arterial PO_2 cannot go above 100 mm Hg while breathing room air at sea level
   d. A continuously negative alveolar–arterial PO_2 difference is incompatible with life
   e. If arterial pH is normal, the patient cannot have a clinically significant acid–base disorder

10. Which of the following statements about noninvasive blood gas monitoring is(are) true?
   a. In the presence of excess carboxyhemoglobin, the pulse oximeter will give a falsely high reading of oxygen saturation

b. The pulse oximeter requires a detectable pulse in order to measure oxygen saturation
c. In the hemodynamically stable patient, the pulse oximeter is equal in accuracy to the co-oximeter
d. The end-tidal PCO_2 is usually equal to or higher than a simultaneously measured $PaCO_2$
e. End-tidal PCO_2 can be used to determine restoration of circulation during cardiopulmonary resuscitation

Quik-Course on Blood Gas Interpretation

INTRODUCTION TO ABG QUIK-COURSE

Chapters 1–8 contain the basics of what most clinicians "really need to know" about blood gases. Problems and self-assessment que+stions are interspersed to help ensure your understanding of the material. Chapters 9–11 are designed to help you "put it all together."

It is possible this amount of information may be more than you really want to study, at least for now. To accommodate those who want to begin with a quick review, or just don't have time to read the whole book right now, I have developed this ABG Quik-Course, an abbreviated syllabus on blood gas interpretation.

ABG Quik-Course includes the four major equations without in-depth explanations and omits all the problems and figures. It is not *all* anyone needs to know, but it is a synopsis of the first eight chapters, and is presented at the beginning so you can use it in a way that best suits your purpose. You can use the ABG Quik-Course as a starting point, as a final review, or as a refresher at any time.

The learning is up to you. Good luck!

FOUR EQUATIONS AND THREE PHYSIOLOGIC PROCESSES (CHAPTERS 1 AND 2)

Arterial blood gas data include both measured and derived values. To obtain the following information, an aliquot of arterial blood is entered into two different machines (or one machine with two distinct components): a blood gas analyzer and a co-oximeter. HCO_3^-, base excess. and arterial oxygen content (CaO_2) are calculations in most blood gas laboratories.

NORMAL ARTERIAL BLOOD GAS VALUES*

pH	7.35–7.45
$PaCO_2$	35–45 mm Hg
PaO_2	70–100 mm Hg†
SaO_2	93–98%
HCO_3^-	22–26 mEq/L
%MetHb	$< 2.0\%$
%COHb	$< 3.0\%$
Base excess	−2.0 to 2.0 mEq/L
CaO_2	16–22 mL O_2/dL

*At sea level, breathing ambient air.
†Age dependent.

Blood gas data provide useful information on three physiologic processes: alveolar ventilation, oxygenation, and acid–base balance. Four equations aid in understanding these processes in the clinical setting:

EQUATION	PHYSIOLOGIC PROCESS
1. $PaCO_2$ equation	Alveolar ventilation
2. Alveolar gas equation	Oxygenation
3. Oxygen content equation	Oxygenation
4. Henderson–Hasselbalch equation	Acid–base balance

1. $PaCO_2$ AND ALVEOLAR VENTILATION (CHAPTER 3)

Alveolar ventilation is the amount of air, in L/min, that reaches the alveoli *and* takes part in gas exchange. Alveolar ventilation is the only process by which the body can excrete the huge amount of CO_2 produced by metabolism. The CO_2 enters tissue capillaries and travels to the lungs where it is excreted in the fresh air brought to the alveoli (the alveolar ventilation). In a steady state, the amount of CO_2 added to the blood equals the amount of CO_2 excreted by the lungs; in a typical resting individual, this is approximately 200 mL CO_2/min.

$PaCO_2$ will go up if CO_2 production exceeds alveolar ventilation and will go down if alveolar ventilation exceeds CO_2 production. $PaCO_2$ is thus directly related to the rate of CO_2 production ($\dot{V}CO_2$) and inversely related to alveolar ventilation ($\dot{V}A$); this very important relationship is reflected in the $PaCO_2$ equation:

$$PaCO_2 = \frac{\dot{V}O_2 \times 0.863}{\dot{V}A}$$

The constant 0.863 converts units for $\dot{V}CO_2$ (mL/min STPD) and $\dot{V}A$ (L/min BTPS) into $PaCO_2$ units of mm Hg. Clinically, it is not necessary to know either $\dot{V}CO_2$ or $\dot{V}A$ but *only their ratio,* which is provided by $PaCO_2$. The following terms characterize high, normal, and low $PaCO_2$ values.

$PaCO_2$ (mm HG)	CONDITION IN BLOOD	STATE OF ALVEOLAR VENTILATION
> 45	Hypercapnia	Hypoventilation
35–45	Eucapnia	Normal ventilation
< 35	Hypocapnia	Hyperventilation

The terms *hypoventilation* and *hyperventilation* should be reserved for specific $PaCO_2$ measurements; they should *not* be used to characterize a patient's rate or depth of breathing, or degree of respiratory effort.

Hypercapnia is a common and serious respiratory problem. The $PaCO_2$ equation shows that the only physiologic reason for elevated $PaCO_2$ is inadequate alveolar ventilation for the amount of CO_2 production. Because alveolar ventilation ($\dot{V}A$) equals total ventilation ($\dot{V}E$) minus dead space ventilation ($\dot{V}D$), hypercapnia can arise from insufficient $\dot{V}E$, increased $\dot{V}D$, or a combination.

Examples of inadequate $\dot{V}E$: sedative drug overdose, respiratory muscle paralysis, central hypoventilation

Examples of increased $\dot{V}D$: chronic obstructive pulmonary disease, severe restrictive lung disease (with shallow, rapid breathing)

The $PaCO_2$ equation shows why $PaCO_2$ cannot reliably be assessed clinically. Because you never know the patient's $\dot{V}CO_2$ or $\dot{V}A$, you cannot determine their ratio, which is what $PaCO_2$ provides.

There is no predictable correlation between $PaCO_2$ and the clinical picture. **Any combination of respiratory rate, depth, or effort can reflect any $PaCO_2$ value, and vice versa.** A patient in profound respiratory distress can have a high, normal, or low $PaCO_2$. A patient with no clinically apparent respiratory problem can have a high, normal, or low $PaCO_2$.

The bedside measurement of total or minute ventilation (tidal volume times respiratory rate) does not give the patient's $\dot{V}CO_2$ or $\dot{V}D$, and so does not provide any information about $\dot{V}A$ or $PaCO_2$. When there is concern about the adequacy of a patient's ventilation, $PaCO_2$ must be measured invasively by arterial blood gas or noninvasively by end-tidal PCO_2. Once PCO_2 is measured, it can be interpreted only in light of the full clinical picture.

Besides indicating a serious derangement in the respiratory system, hypercapnia poses a threat to the patient for three reasons:

- An increased $PaCO_2$ will lower the PAO_2 (equation 2)
- An increased $PaCO_2$ will lower the pH (equation 4)
- The higher the baseline $PaCO_2$, the greater it will rise for a given fall in $\dot{V}A$ (e.g., a 1 L/min decrease in $\dot{V}A$ will raise $PaCO_2$ a greater amount when the baseline is 50 mm Hg than when it is 40 mm Hg).

$PaCO_2$ is a component of formulas that help determine both oxygenation and acid–base status: the alveolar gas equation for alveolar PO_2 and the Henderson–Hasselbalch equation for pH. Both equations are discussed in the sections that follow.

2. PaO_2, PAO_2 AND THE ALVEOLAR GAS EQUATION (CHAPTER 4)

PaO_2 is the partial pressure of oxygen in arterial blood, measured in mm Hg (or torr; 1 mm Hg = 1 torr). PaO_2 does not reveal how much oxygen is in the blood (see Chapters 5 and 6) but only the pressure exerted by dissolved (unbound) O_2 molecules against the measuring electrode. PaO_2 is usually reduced in the presence of ventilation–perfusion (V–Q) imbalance, the physiologic state characteristic of many airway and alveolar disease processes (e.g., asthma, atelectasis, bronchitis, pneumonia, pulmonary edema, pulmonary embolism).

The *upper* limit of PaO_2 is determined by the mean alveolar PO_2 (PAO_2). In a steady state, the measured PaO_2 cannot be higher than the calculated PAO_2; a continuously negative A–a PO_2 difference is incompatible with life. The *lower* limit of PaO_2 is determined by several factors but principally by the extent of the V–Q imbalance. Normal PaO_2 is age dependent; breathing room air, at sea level, PaO_2 ranges from a high of 100 mm Hg in children down to the 70s in octogenarians: $PaO_2 = 109 - 0.43(\text{age in years})$. The normal decline of PaO_2 with age is due largely to natural loss of lung compliance, which causes a worsening of the ventilation–perfusion imbalance.

Whereas PaO_2 is a laboratory measurement, PAO_2 is a calculation derived from the alveolar gas equation. In essence, PAO_2 equals the inspired PO_2 (PIO_2) minus the alveolar PCO_2 ($PaCO_2$) times 1.2. Because $PaCO_2$ is assumed equal to $PaCO_2$, the latter is used in the abbreviated form of the alveolar gas equation:

$$PAO_2 = PIO_2 - 1.2\ (PaCO_2)$$

where

$$PIO_2 = FIO_2\ (P_B - 47)$$

PIO_2 is a function of the FIO_2 and barometric pressure; 47 mm Hg is the water vapor pressure at normal body temperature, and must be subtracted from P_B. Unlike PaO_2, PAO_2 is not age dependent but remains constant so long as the variables in the equation are unchanged.

Are the lungs transferring oxygen properly? The answer is found by the *difference* between calculated PAO_2 and measured PaO_2. This difference, $P(A\text{–}a)O_2$, is colloquially called the *A–a gradient,* although it does not reflect a true gradient but rather a state of ventilation–perfusion imbalance within the lungs. The range for normal $P(A\text{–}a)O_2$ increases with age and FIO_2. When $FIO_2 = 1.00$, normal $P(A\text{–}a)O_2$ can range up to 110 mm Hg.

Without knowledge of PAO_2 one cannot properly interpret any PaO_2 value. Is a PaO_2 of 90 mm Hg normal? A PaO_2 of 28 mm Hg abnormal? You must know the variables in the alveolar gas equation to clinically interpret any PaO_2 value. A PaO_2 of 90 mm Hg is normal in a subject with normal $PaCO_2$ breathing room air at sea level. The same PaO_2 is abnormal if $PaCO_2$ is 25 mm Hg; the alveolar gas equation shows that the PAO_2 (and hence the PaO_2) should be about 15 mm Hg higher, i.e., $PAO_2 = 120$ mm Hg and $PaO_2 = 105$ mm Hg. A PaO_2 of 90 mm Hg would also be abnormal—and indicate severely impaired lungs—in a patient breathing 100% oxygen at sea level. Under these conditions, PAO_2 should be over 600 mm Hg with normal lungs, and PaO_2 at least 500 mm Hg.

In terms of oxygen transfer, a PaO_2 of 28 mm Hg would be normal on the summit of Mount Everest (29,028 ft.) for a climber breathing pure mountain air. Barometric pressure at this altitude has been measured at only 253 mm Hg; with extreme hyperventilation (to 7.5 mm Hg PCO2), the resulting PAO_2 and PaO_2 were estimated at only 35 and 28 mm Hg, respectively. A PaO_2 of 28 mm Hg would also be normal in someone inhaling only 8% oxygen. The subject in either situation is *hypoxemic,* but not because of any lung disease or defect in oxygen transfer.

In summary, PaO_2 must always be interpreted with knowledge of the $PaCO_2$, FIO_2, and barometric pressure, variables that are incorporated into the alveolar gas equation for PAO_2. A low PaO_2 with increased $P(A\text{–}a)O_2$ points to ventilation–perfusion imbalance and disease within the lungs. The vast majority of patients with low PaO_2 have ventilation–perfusion imbalance and so manifest an increased $P(A\text{–}a)O_2$. The following table lists this and other physiologic causes of a low PaO_2 and elevated $P(A\text{–}a)O_2$.

CAUSES OF LOW PaO_2	$P(A-a)O_2$
Nonrespiratory	
Cardiac right-to-left shunt	Increased
Decreased PIO_2	Normal
Low mixed venous oxygen content	Increased
Respiratory	
Pulmonary right-to-left shunt	Increased
Ventilation–perfusion imbalance	Increased
Diffusion barrier	Increased
Hypoventilation (increased $PaCO_2$)	Normal

3. SaO_2 and oxygen content (Chapters 5 and 6)

Tissues need a requisite amount of oxygen molecules for metabolism. Neither the PaO_2 nor the SaO_2 tells *how much* oxygen is in the blood. *How much* is provided by the oxygen content, CaO_2 (units ml O_2/dl). CaO_2 is calculated as:

$$CaO_2 = \text{quantity } O_2 \text{ bound to hemoglobin} + \text{quantity } O_2 \text{ dissolved in plasma}$$
$$CaO_2 = (Hb \times 1.34 \times SaO_2) + (0.003 \times PaO_2)$$

The quantity of oxygen bound to hemoglobin is the product of the hemoglobin content (Hb, in g/dL), the oxygen carrying capacity of Hb (1.34 mL O_2/g Hb), and the oxygen saturation of Hb in arterial blood (SaO_2). The quantity of oxygen dissolved in plasma is the product of its solubility constant (0.003 mL O_2/dL/mm Hg) and the PaO_2 in mm Hg.

PaO_2, SaO_2, and CaO_2 represent different aspects of oxygenation. PaO_2 depends on PAO_2 and the alveolar–capillary interface; it represents the dissolved fraction of oxygen in plasma and does not depend on the content or nature of hemoglobin. SaO_2 is a function of PaO_2 and the position of the oxygen dissociation curve; the curve's position depends on temperature, pH , $PaCO_2$, and 2,3-DPG. CaO_2 is a function of SaO_2, hemoglobin content, and to a lesser extent, the PaO_2.

Hypoxemia can be broadly defined as low oxygen in the blood and more specifically as a reduced PaO_2, SaO_2, *and/or* CaO_2. *Hypoxia* is a more general term than hypoxemia; it signifies reduced oxygen to the body as a whole and includes all causes of hypoxemia.

Causes of hypoxia—a general classification

1. Hypoxemia
   a. Reduced PaO_2—most commonly from lung disease (most common physiologic mechanism: V–Q imbalance)

   b. Reduced SaO_2—most commonly from reduced PaO_2; other causes include carbon monoxide poisoning, methemoglobinemia, or rightward shift of the O_2 dissociation curve
   c. Reduced hemoglobin content—anemia
2. Reduced oxygen delivery to the tissues
   a. Reduced cardiac output—shock, congestive heart failure
   b. Left-to-right systemic shunt (as may be seen in septic shock)
3. Decreased tissue oxygen uptake
   a. Mitochondrial poisoning (e.g., cyanide poisoning)
   b. Left-shifted hemoglobin dissociation curve (e.g., from acute alkalosis, excess CO, or abnormal hemoglobin structure)

Carboxyhemoglobin

Every blood gas lab measures PaO_2 but not all measure SaO_2; some labs calculate SaO_2 based on the PaO_2 and a standard oxygen dissociation curve (adjusted for the patient's measured pH and temperature). A calculated SaO_2 is potentially misleading as it will miss two important causes of hypoxemia that lower SaO_2 without affecting PaO_2: carbon monoxide poisoning and methemoglobinemia.

Carbon monoxide is a colorless, odorless gas that results from incomplete combustion of hydrocarbon fuels. It causes hypoxemia two ways. First, CO displaces O_2 from hemoglobin to form carboxyhemoglobin (COHb) and thereby reduces the SaO_2 and oxygen content. Second, CO shifts the oxygen dissociation curve *to the left*. As a result of the left shift, oxygen that is taken up by hemoglobin is held *more tightly than normal*, making less O_2 available to the tissues for any given PO_2 value.

Normal COHb is $< 3\%$ in urban dwellers. Between 5 and 10% COHb is commonly found in cigarette and cigar smokers. Symptoms begin at higher values, with coma and death occurring above 50% COHb. Excess COHb should always be suspected if the *measured* SaO_2 is significantly lower than predicted for the PaO_2 (e.g., $PaO_2 = 80$ mm Hg with a measured SaO_2 of 85%). The diagnosis is confirmed by direct measurement of %COHb. Co-oximeters can measure both SaO_2 and %COHb. Also, note that COHb can be measured in venous blood, so an arterial sample is not necessary to make the diagnosis of carbon monoxide poisoning.

Note that pulse oximeters *do not* distinguish between oxyhemoglobin and carboxyhemoglobin and so cannot be used to detect carbon monoxide excess. A patient with 30% COHb and a true (if measured with a co-oximeter) SaO_2 of 65% will have a pulse oximeter oxygen saturation of 95%.

Methemoglobin

Normal hemoglobin contains iron in the ferrous or Fe^{++} state. It is in this state that hemoglobin binds to oxygen in the pulmonary capillaries. Methemoglobin contains iron in the ferric (oxidized) or Fe^{+++} state, which makes the hemoglobin unable to bind oxygen. This oxidized hemoglobin state is usually caused by a drug reaction (to nitrates, topical anesthetics, etc.) and is reversible with time (severe cases are treated with the reducing agent methylene blue). Like COHb, excess methemoglobin does not lower PaO_2 but only SaO_2. Methemoglobin can be directly measured by a co-oximeter, or suspected by the presence of intense cyanosis in a patient with normal PaO_2. Unlike CO, excess methemoglobin depresses the pulse oximeter reading of SaO_2 somewhat, but not linearly (see Chapter 6 for further discussion of this topic).

4. ACID–BASE BALANCE (CHAPTERS 7 AND 8)

The concentration of hydrogen ion is related to the concentration of carbonic acid and bicarbonate. The Henderson–Hasselbalch equation defines the hydrogen ion concentration in terms of pH as follows:

$$pH = pK + \log \frac{[HCO_3^-]}{0.03\ [PaCO_2]}$$

pH is a confusing term for acidity, because small numerical changes represent large and *opposite* changes in hydrogen ion concentration $[H^+]$. A pH change of 1.00 represents a 10-fold change in $[H^+]$. Thus

pH	$[H^+]$ (nMol/L)
7.00	100
7.10	80
7.30	50
7.40	40
7.52	30
7.70	20
8.00	10

Clinical and physiologic acid–base disorders do not always lead to predictable changes in the blood. Any given set of blood gases (e.g., low pH, low $PaCO_2$, low HCO_3^-) can come from several pathways and represent many different clinical disorders. By convention, terms ending in *-emia* apply to blood changes only; terms ending in *-osis* apply to physiologic processes that may or may not lead to particular changes in the blood. The following terminology is now widely accepted in describing and discussing acid–base disorders.

Acidemia: Blood pH < 7.35

Acidosis: A primary physiologic process that, occurring alone, tends to cause acidemia, e.g., metabolic acidosis from decreased perfusion (lactic acidosis); respiratory acidosis from hypoventilation. If the patient has an alkalosis at the same time, the resulting blood pH may be low, normal, or high.

Alkalemia: Blood pH > 7.45

Alkalosis: A primary physiologic process that, occurring alone, tends to cause alkalemia. Examples: metabolic alkalosis from excessive diuretic therapy and respiratory alkalosis from acute hyperventilation. If the patient has an acidosis at the same time, the resulting blood pH may be high, normal, or low.

Primary acid–base disorder: One of the four acid–base disturbances that is manifested by an initial change in HCO_3^- or $PaCO_2$. If HCO_3^- changes first, the disorder is either a metabolic acidosis (reduced HCO_3^- and acidemia) or metabolic alkalosis (elevated HCO_3^- and alkalemia). If $PaCO_2$ changes first, the problem is either respiratory alkalosis (reduced $PaCO_2$ and alkalemia) or respiratory acidosis (elevated $PaCO_2$ and acidemia).

Compensation: The change in HCO_3^- or $PaCO_2$ that results from the primary event. Compensatory changes are not classified by the terms used for the four primary acid–base disturbances. For example, a patient who hyperventilates (lowers $PaCO_2$) solely as compensation for metabolic acidosis does *not* have a respiratory alkalosis, the latter being a primary disorder that, alone, would lead to alkalemia. In simple, uncomplicated metabolic acidosis the patient will never develop alkalemia.

Primary acid–base disorders

The four primary acid–base disorders are defined below; some clinical causes for each are listed on page xxxiii.

Respiratory alkalosis: A disorder in which the first change is a lowering of $PaCO_2$, resulting in an elevated pH. Compensation is a secondary lowering of bicarbonate by the kidneys; this reduction in HCO_3^- is not metabolic acidosis, since it is not a primary process.

Respiratory acidosis: A disorder in which the first change is an elevation of $PaCO_2$, resulting in decreased pH. Compensation is a secondary retention of bicarbonate by the kidneys; this elevation of HCO_3^- is not metabolic alkalosis, because it is not a primary process.

Metabolic acidosis: A disorder in which the first change is a lowering of HCO_3^-, resulting in decreased pH. Compensation is a secondary hyperventilation; this lowering of $PaCO_2$ is not respiratory alkalosis, because it is not a primary process. Metabolic acidosis is conveniently divided into elevated and normal anion gap acidosis. Anion gap (AG) is calculated as

$$AG = Na^+ - (Cl^- + CO_2)$$

CO_2 in this equation is the "total CO_2" measured in the chemistry lab as part of routine serum electrolytes and consists mostly of bicarbonate. The normal AG calculated in this manner is 12 ± 4 mEq/L. If AG is calculated using K^+, the normal gap is 16 ± 4 mEq/L. (Normal values for AG may vary among labs, so one should always refer to local normal values before making clinical decisions based on the AG.)

High anion gap acidosis arises from excess acid added to the blood that has an unmeasured anion, e.g., lactic acidosis (lactate anion). Metabolic acidosis with a normal AG occurs one of two ways: when the excess acid that is added to the blood contains chloride as the anion (since this is measured) and from loss of bicarbonate by the kidneys or gastrointestinal (GI) system.

Metabolic alkalosis: A disorder in which the first change is an elevation of HCO_3^-, resulting in increased pH. Metabolic alkalosis can occur from excess bicarbonate added to the blood or from loss of HCl. The former can occur from administration of alkali or from excess renal reabsorption HCO_3^- (common with diuretic therapy). GI loss of HCl is common with nasogastric suctioning and vomiting. Compensation is a secondary hypoventilation (increased $PaCO_2$), which is not respiratory acidosis, since it is not a primary process. Compensation for metabolic alkalosis is less predictable than for the other three acid–base disorders (see Chapter 8 for further discussion).

Some clinical causes of the four primary acid–base disorders

Metabolic acidosis

Increased anion gap: lactic acidosis, ketoacidosis, drug poisonings (aspirin, ethylene glycol, methanol)

Normal anion gap: diarrhea, some kidney problems (renal tubular acidosis, interstitial nephritis)

Metabolic alkalosis

Chloride responsive, i.e., responds to NaCl or KCl therapy (contraction alkalosis, diuretics, corticosteroids, gastric suctioning, vomiting)

Chloride resistant: any hyperaldosterone state (Cushing syndrome, Bartter syndrome, severe K^+ depletion)

Respiratory acidosis (= respiratory failure)

Central nervous system depression (drug overdose)

Chest bellows dysfunction (Guillain-Barré syndrome, myasthenia gravis)

Disease of lungs and/or upper airway (chronic obstructive lung disease, severe asthma attack, severe pulmonary edema)

Respiratory alkalosis

Hypoxemia (includes altitude)

Anxiety

Sepsis

Any acute pulmonary insult (pneumonia, mild asthma attack, early pulmonary edema, pulmonary embolism)

TIPS FOR DIAGNOSING MIXED ACID–BASE DISORDERS

Often there is more than one acid–base disorder in the same patient at the same time. The following observations are useful for diagnosing mixed acid–base disorders.

TIP 1. Don't interpret any blood gas data for acid–base diagnosis without closely examining the serum electrolytes: Na^+, K^+, Cl^-, and CO_2.

- A serum CO_2 out of the normal range always represents some type of acid–base disorder (barring lab or transcription error).

  High serum CO_2 = metabolic alkalosis and/or bicarbonate retention as compensation for respiratory acidosis

  Low serum CO_2 = metabolic acidosis and/or bicarbonate excretion as compensation for respiratory alkalosis

  Note that serum CO_2 may be normal in the presence of two or more acid–base disorders.

- Calculate the anion gap (AG) as discussed under "Metabolic Acidosis." If AG $\geq$ 20 mEq/L, the patient likely has an anion gap metabolic acidosis (see the causes, above).
- If AG is elevated, calculate the bicarbonate gap (BG):

$$BG = \Delta AG - \Delta CO_2 = (AG - 12) - (27 - CO_2)$$

which can be reduced to the following shortcut:

$$BG = Na^+ - Cl^- - 39$$

- There is no agreed on normal range for BG, but a value outside of $\pm$ 6 mEq/L strongly suggests that CO_2 is out of line for the elevated AG and there is likely another acid–base disorder. Thus

$BG > +6$ mEq/L = metabolic alkalosis and/or bicarbonate retention as compensation for respiratory acidosis (same as for high serum CO_2)
$BG < -6$ mEq/L = hyperchloremic metabolic acidosis and/or bicar = bonate excretion as compensation for respiratory alkalosis

TIP 2. Single acid–base disorders do not lead to normal blood pH. Although pH can end up in the normal range (7.35–7.45) with single disorders of a mild degree, a truly normal pH with distinctly abnormal HCO_3^- or $PaCO_2$ invariably suggests two or more primary disorders. Example: pH = 7.40, $PaCO_2$ = 20 mm Hg, HCO_3^- = 12 mEq/L, in a patient with sepsis. His normal pH resulted from two co-existing and unstable acid–base disorders: acute respiratory alkalosis and metabolic acidosis.

TIP 3. Simplified rules predict the pH and HCO_3^- for a given change in $PaCO_2$. If the pH or HCO_3^- is higher or lower than expected for the change in $PaCO_2$, the patient probably has a metabolic acid–base disorder as well. The rules below show the expected changes in pH and HCO_3^- (in mEq/L) for *a 10 mm Hg change* in $PaCO_2$ from either primary hypoventilation (respiratory acidosis) or primary hyperventilation (respiratory alkalosis).

CONDITION	ACUTE	CHRONIC
Respiratory acidosis	pH ↓ by 0.07 HCO_3^- ↑ by 1	pH ↓ by 0.03 HCO_3^- ↑ by 3–4
Respiratory alkalosis	pH ↑ by 0.08 HCO_3^- ↓ by 2	pH ↑ by 0.03 HCO_3^- ↓ by 5

These rules are quite useful in diagnosing a mixed acid–base disorder when there is respiratory acidosis or respiratory alkalosis. Acute CO_2 retention (i.e., acute hypoventilation) drives the hydration reaction (shown in Chapter 7) to the right; as a result, HCO_3^- increases slightly. Acute CO_2

excretion (i.e., acute hyperventilation) drives the hydration equation to the left, and HCO_3^- decreases slightly. These changes in HCO_3^- are instantaneous and have *nothing* to do with the kidneys or renal compensation. Thus

- A normal or slightly low HCO_3^- in the presence of hypercapnia suggests a concomitant metabolic acidosis, e.g., pH = 7.27, $PaCO_2$ = 50 mm Hg, and HCO_3^- = 22 mEq/L
- A normal or slightly elevated HCO_3^- in the presence of hypocapnia suggests a concomitant metabolic alkalosis, e.g., pH = 7.56, $PaCO_2$ = 30 mm Hg, and HCO_3^- 26 mEq/L.

TIP 4. In maximally compensated metabolic acidosis, the numerical value of $PaCO_2$ should be the same (or close to) the last two digits of arterial pH. This observation reflects the following formula for the expected respiratory compensation in metabolic acidosis:

$$\text{Expected } PaCO_2 = [1.5 \times \text{serum } CO_2] + (8 \pm 2)$$

In contrast, compensation for metabolic alkalosis (by increase in $PaCO_2$) is highly variable, and in some cases there may be no or minimal increases in $PaCO_2$.

SUMMARY—CLINICAL AND LABORATORY APPROACH TO ACID–BASE DIAGNOSIS

- Determine existence of acid–base disorder from arterial blood gas and/or serum electrolyte measurements. Check serum CO_2; if abnormal there is an acid–base disorder. If the anion gap is significantly increased there is a metabolic acidosis. If bicarbonate gap significantly deviates from zero there is an additional acid–base disorder besides anion gap acidosis.
- Examine pH, $PaCO_2$, and HCO_3^- for the obvious primary acid–base disorder, and for deviations that indicate mixed acid–base disorders (Tips 2–4).
- Use a full clinical assessment (history, physical exam, other lab data including previous arterial blood gases and serum electrolytes) to explain each acid–base disorder (see the chart, above). Remember that coexisting clinical conditions may lead to opposing acid–base disorders, so that pH can be high when there is an obvious acidosis, or low when there is an obvious alkalosis.
- Treat the underlying clinical condition(s); this will usually suffice to correct most acid–base disorders. If there is concern that acidemia or alkalemia is life-threatening, aim toward correcting pH into the range of 7.30–7.52 ($[H^+]$ = 50–30 nMol/L).
- **Clinical judgment should always apply.**

CHAPTER

1

What Is Meant by Interpreting Arterial Blood Gases?

One Blood Sample, Two Sets of Tests

ONE BLOOD SAMPLE

This book is about how to interpret and use lab values obtained from a single arterial blood sample. Usually obtained from a radial, brachial, or femoral artery, the blood is brought to the lab in a heparinized, ice-encased syringe, where it is promptly tested. Turnaround time from arterial blood drawing to results reporting is typically 10–20 min.

Strictly speaking, *blood gas* refers to any element or compound that is a gas under ordinary conditions and that is also dissolved to some extent in our blood. With this definition in mind, circle any of the following values that represent *blood gases*. The terms are listed in alphabetical order. (Please make sure you circle your answers before reading further.)

a. Base excess
b. Bicarbonate
c. Carbon dioxide
d. Carbon monoxide
e. Glucose
f. Helium
g. Hemoglobin
h. Krypton
i. Nitrogen
j. Oxygen
k. pH

Carbon dioxide, carbon monoxide, helium, krypton, nitrogen, and oxygen are gases under ordinary conditions and are also dissolved in our blood, hence they are all blood gases. Although pH is not a gas, it is routinely measured with arterial blood gases (ABG) and is now firmly fixed as part the *ABG test.* Similarly, bicarbonate, not a blood gas but the anion of carbonic acid, is routinely calculated as part of every blood gas test. Base excess is a calculation that reflects how much acid or base is needed to normalize the total buffer base in the blood (see Chapter 7).

Although glucose is also dissolved in blood, it is not a gas but a granular material at room temperature. Similarly, hemoglobin, the molecular carrier of oxygen within the red blood cell, is not a gas under any condition.

Nitrogen, krypton, and helium are inert gases dissolved in our blood (the last two in trace amounts). Because inert gases cause no clinical problems, they are not measured as part of the arterial blood gas test. (Nitrogen can cause the bends and other problems in compressed air diving, but this is a highly specialized area of medicine and the problems are not diagnosed with blood gas measurements.)

Carbon monoxide *is* a gas and is measured in its combined form with hemoglobin as percent carboxyhemoglobin (%COHb). Thus a value of 10% carboxyhemoglobin means that 10% of the potential oxygen-binding sites on hemoglobin are occupied by CO. Carbon monoxide *could* be measured in its dissolved state (as partial pressure of CO), but this component is minute, and its measurement is only an indirect guide to the %COHb. So %COHb is what the blood gas lab is set up to measure.

In summary, not all blood gases are routinely measured and not all blood gas measurements are of true blood gases. Carbon dioxide and oxygen are routinely measured as their partial pressures, $PaCO_2$ and PaO_2, respectively. Carbon monoxide, another blood gas, is measured as %COHb. Nitrogen, helium, and krypton (as well as other inert blood gases) are not measured at all.

TWO SETS OF TESTS

All blood gas labs have a machine to measure pH, $PaCO_2$, and PaO_2 and to calculate (or allow for calculation of) the bicarbonate value. In addition, *many but not all* labs also have a machine called a co-oximeter (Fig. 1.1).

The co-oximeter can measure, on a small portion of the arterial blood sample, hemoglobin content (in grams per deciliter) and values related to hemoglobin binding: SaO_2, %COHb, and percent methemoglobin (%MetHb). From this information, the arterial oxygen content (CaO_2) can be calculated.

The one- versus two-machine arrangement is the case in most labs. However, newer technology now incorporates both machines within a single console, so that both sets of measurements (blood gases per se, and co-oximetry measurements) can be made from a single entered sample (Fig. 1.2).

Why do I emphasize *two machines* and *two sets of measurements*? The answer is that many people who routinely interpret arterial blood gases are un-

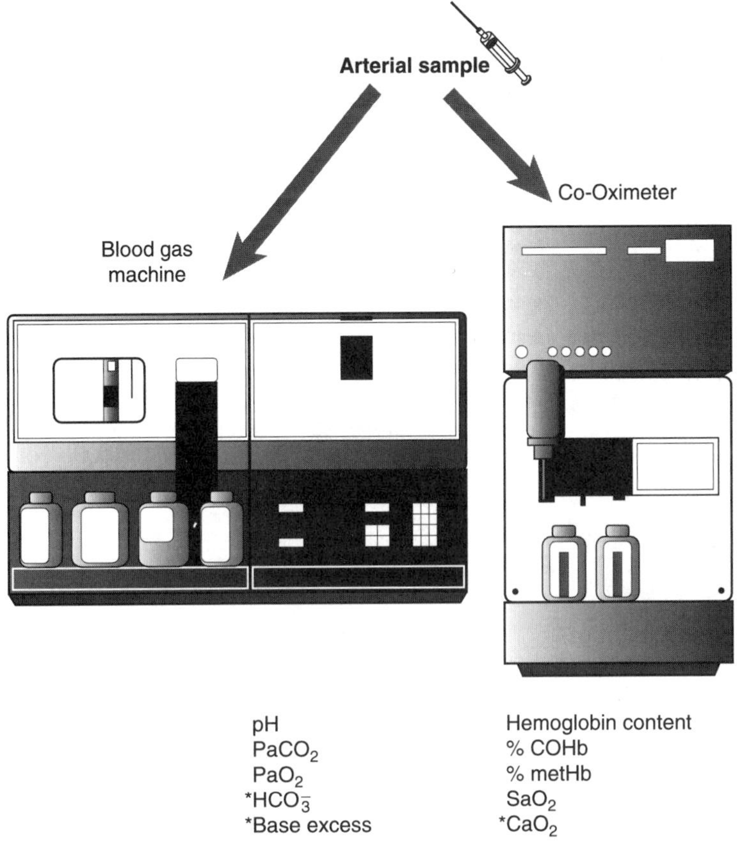

Figure 1.1. Two blood gas machines: measurements and calculations (*).

aware of the fact that co-oximetry is a distinct test that (*a*) may not be available or (*b*) if available, may not be run because it wasn't specifically ordered by the physician.

If co-oximetry is not available or is available and not ordered, one can miss such life-threatening conditions as carbon monoxide poisoning and methemoglobinemia. In these conditions the PaO_2 is normal unless the patient has co-existing lung disease; furthermore, the SaO_2 value calculated from the PaO_2 will be falsely high, thus setting the stage for possible serious misdiagnosis (see Chapter 6).

Whatever the arrangement in your particular lab, it is important to keep in mind that a complete "blood gas analysis" involves two sets of measurements: blood gases and measurements related to hemoglobin content and binding.

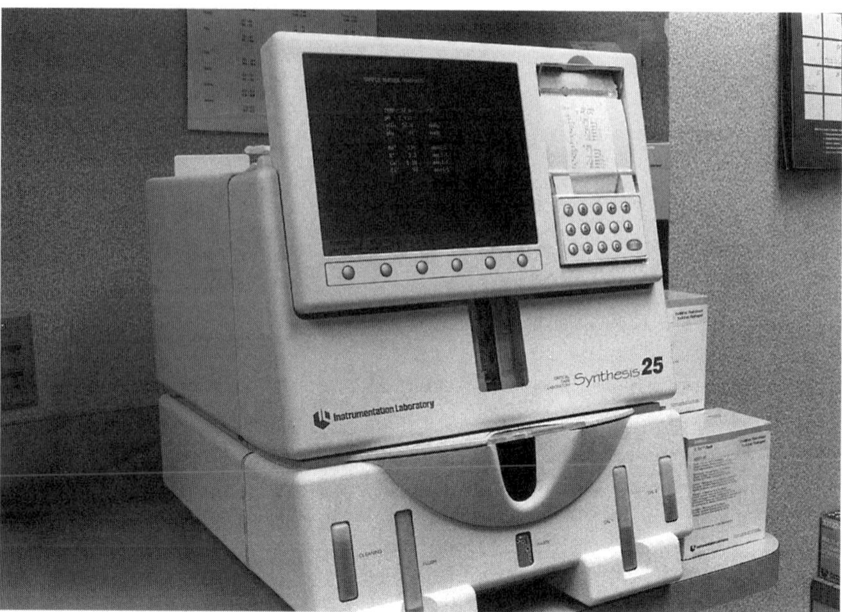

Figure 1.2. An analyzer console that incorporates both a blood gas machine and a co-oximeter. From a single aliquot of blood, one can obtain all the information shown in Table 1.1.

The three types of *machine arrangements* found in blood gas labs can be summarized as follows:

- A blood gas machine only. These labs cannot do co-oximetry (hemoglobin-related) measurements.
- A blood gas machine and a separate co-oximeter (Fig. 1.1). The arterial sample is divided between the two machines for a complete blood gas analysis.
- A single machine that incorporates blood gas and co-oximetry measurements from a single sample (Fig. 1.2).

On the lines below, write the machine arrangement in your blood gas lab and state what you have to do to obtain co-oximetry measurements on any arterial blood sample (Is it routinely done? Does it require a separate lab slip?, etc.).

This is one question I can't answer for you. I recommend you find out the answers and not let it pass.

Now, for a question we can answer together: What is the maximum value attainable by adding the values obtained for SaO_2, %COHb, and %MetHb from a single blood sample?

a. 100%
b. 200%
c. Depends on the hemoglobin content

Just as %COHb is the percent of hemoglobin sites chemically combined with carbon monoxide, SaO_2 is the percentage of hemoglobin sites chemically combined (*saturated*) with oxygen, i.e., the $\%O_2Hb$ (SaO_2 seems to be the more popular term). A hemoglobin-binding site cannot contain more than one gas molecule at the same time, so the two percentages ($\%O_2Hb$ and %COHb) are additive.

Methemoglobin is hemoglobin that has iron in its ferric or oxidized state (Fe^{+++}) as opposed to the normal ferrous state (Fe^{++}); hemoglobin with Fe^{+++} can bind *neither* oxygen *nor* carbon monoxide. Thus SaO_2, %COHb, and %MetHb each represent separate portions of the total hemoglobin content and together cannot exceed 100%.

In summary, the blood gas machine is used to measure partial pressure of oxygen and carbon dioxide (PO_2 and PCO_2) and pH, and to perform some calculations based on these data. The co-oximeter (either a separate machine or incorporated into the blood gas machine) is used to measure the quantity and various states of hemoglobin, values that allow for calculation of oxygen content (see Chapter 2). All blood gas labs are set up to measure PO_2, PCO_2, and pH; many labs also run the arterial sample through a co-oximeter to measure additional values (Figs. 1.1 and 1.2). Normal values for blood gas measurements and calculations are shown in Table 1.1.

ELECTROLYTE MEASUREMENTS

Over the past decade, many blood gas labs have taken on an additional task: measuring electrolytes in the arterial sample (sodium, potassium, chloride, bicarbonate, and occasionally calcium and magnesium). This has been made possible by incorporating special electrodes into the blood gas machine. The model shown in Figure 1.2 can measure electrolytes in the same arterial sam-

TABLE 1.1. NORMAL ARTERIAL BLOOD GAS VALUES[a]

MEASUREMENT	VALUE
pH	7.35–7.45
$PaCO_2$	35–45 mm Hg
PaO_2	> 70 mm Hg[b]
HCO_3^-	22–26 mEq/L
SaO_2	93–98%[b]
%MetHb	< 2%
%COHb	< 3.0%
Base excess	−2.0 to 2.0 mEq/L
CaO_2	16–22 mL O_2/dL

[a]At sea level, breathing ambient air.
[b]Age-dependent.

ple used for blood gas and co-oximetry measurements. Electrolytes as an aid to acid–base diagnosis are discussed in Chapter 7.

HOW MUCH PHYSIOLOGY DO YOU NEED TO KNOW FOR PROPER BLOOD GAS INTERPRETATION?

No doubt about it, a knowledge of some basic pulmonary physiology is crucial to understanding arterial blood gas data. The next chapter introduces the three physiologic processes and four equations important in blood gas interpretation.

Physiology textbooks teach the basics, but most of them don't relate the material to specific blood gas data or the clinical setting. Without the basics, however, you cannot build any clinical understanding. If you have a standard physiology textbook, you might want to review the sections on oxygenation, ventilation, and acid–base balance as you work through this book. Texts particularly recommended for such review (if needed) are listed in Appendix E: Bibliography. *All You Really Need to Know to Interpret Arterial Blood Gases* is predicated on basic physiology as taught in medical school and in all respiratory therapy and 4-year nursing schools. You are the best judge of whether additional review is necessary.

WHAT OTHER INFORMATION IS NEEDED TO INTERPRET BLOOD GAS DATA?

In large part, this book is about how to integrate blood gas values *with additional information,* to intelligently assess alveolar ventilation, oxygenation, and acid–base balance. When you can do that you will have learned to properly interpret blood gas data. In addition to some knowledge of basic pulmonary physiology, three areas of information are necessary for proper blood gas interpretation.

1. Information about the patient's immediate environment:
   - Inspired oxygen (FIO_2)
   - Barometric pressure
2. Additional lab data, for example:
   - Previous blood gas measurements
   - Electrolytes, blood sugar, blood urea nitrogen (BUN)
   - Hemoglobin content or hematocrit
   - Chest x-ray
   - Pulmonary function tests
3. Clinical information, including the history and physical exam, with emphasis on the patient's
   - Respiratory rate and other vital signs
   - Degree of respiratory effort
   - Mental status
   - State of tissue perfusion

When confronted with isolated blood gas data, always ask yourself: **Do I have the necessary clinical and laboratory information to properly interpret these data?**

An isolated $PaCO_2$ reveals little useful information without reference to the patient's mental status and respiratory effort. A low PaO_2 may mean one thing if the patient is inhaling supplemental oxygen and quite another if the patient is breathing room air. Similarly, knowledge of the chest x-ray may be crucial to interpreting a low PaO_2. The pH and HCO_3^- sometimes make sense only in light of the serum electrolytes. To properly interpret blood gas data, you must know the full clinical and laboratory picture.

THE PATIENT'S ENVIRONMENT: FIO_2 AND BAROMETRIC PRESSURE

The value for normal PaO_2 depends on FIO_2, barometric pressure, and the patient's age. Air consists of a mixture of gases, containing approximately 21% oxygen, 78% nitrogen, and 1% other inert gases, a composition that is unchanged throughout the breathable atmosphere. At any altitude, the fraction of inspired oxygen (FIO_2) is 0.21. (FIO_2 is sometimes written as a percentage, e.g., 21%. Either format is acceptable.)

Barometric pressure is a function of the weight of the atmosphere above the point of measurement. At sea level, the barometric pressure averages 760 mm Hg, i.e., air pressure at sea level will sustain a closed column of mercury 760 mm high. The higher the altitude, the lower the weight of air at that point and the lower the barometric pressure. At the highest point on earth, the summit of Mount Everest, the barometric pressure is only 253 mm Hg (Fig. 1.3).

Barometric pressure is the sum of the pressures of all the constituent gases. Each gas exerts its own *partial pressure,* which is the pressure it would exert if no other gases were present. Table 1.2 shows the partial pressures for gases in dry air at sea level.

The partial pressure of any gas in dry air is the percentage of gas in the air times the barometric pressure:

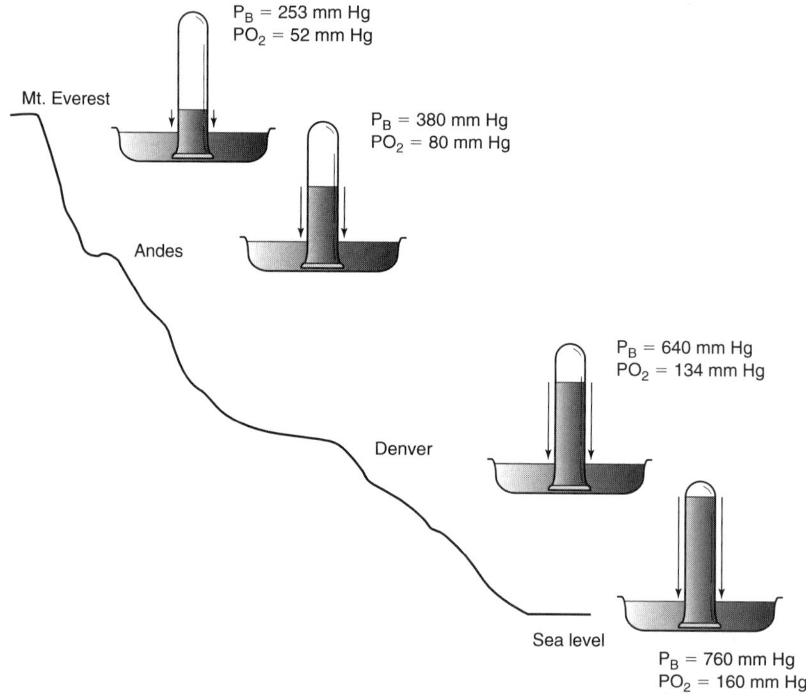

Figure 1.3. Effects of altitude on barometric pressure (P_B). The height of the column of mercury supported by air decreases with increasing altitude owing to the fall in P_B. Here, PO_2 is the partial pressure of oxygen in dry air. Since $PO_2 = 0.21 \times P_B$, PO_2 also decreases with altitude.

TABLE 1.2. COMPOSITION OF DRY AIR AT SEA LEVEL

GAS	PERCENT IN AIR	PARTIAL PRESSURE (mm Hg)
Nitrogen	78.08	593.41
Oxygen	20.95	159.22
Carbon dioxide	00.03	0.23
Other gases[a]	00.94	7.14
Total	100.00	760.00

[a]Mainly argon.

$$P_{GAS} \text{ in dry air} = \text{percentage of gas} \times P_B$$

Why *dry* air? Air often contains water vapor, which exerts its own partial pressure. To obtain the partial pressure of any gas, such as oxygen or nitrogen, water vapor pressure must first be subtracted from the barometric pressure, since it dilutes out all the dry gases. Depending on the climate, the amount of water vapor in ambient air varies from 0 to fully saturated and the partial pressure of water vapor, from 0 to > 50 mm Hg. For example, if ambient air is partly saturated so that P_{H_2O} is 27 mm Hg, then

$$P_{GAS} = \text{percentage of gas} \times (P_B - 27)$$

Regardless of the P_{H_2O} in ambient air, once air is inhaled it becomes fully saturated in the upper airway; hence all *inspired* air has a water vapor pressure of 47 mm Hg (at 98.6°F or 37°C; water vapor pressure varies slightly with body temperature). For this reason, knowledge of the ambient air P_{H_2O} is not clinically important.

Table 1.2 lists the major gases in air and their partial pressures in dry air. Note that for clinical purposes, we round off the percentage of oxygen in the air to 0.21 (21%); this is the FIO_2 (fraction of inspired oxygen) when breathing ambient, or room, air. (Although there is a tiny amount of CO_2 in the atmosphere, for clinical purposes we assume an inspired PCO_2 of 0.)

Since the percentage of oxygen is constant throughout the breathable atmosphere, but the barometric pressure decreases with altitude, the pressure of oxygen must fall with altitude (Fig. 1.2). To maintain acceptable oxygen levels at extreme altitude, there are two broad options: change the environment or adapt physiologically.

The first option involves increasing either the FIO_2 or the barometric pressure. Airplane cabins are pressurized to 7000–8000 feet whenever planes fly much higher than those altitudes; this pressurization allows the FIO_2 to be kept at 0.21 throughout the flight. Pressurization is, of course, not feasible out in the open. Mountain climbers carry portable oxygen to increase their FIO_2 at extreme altitudes (e.g., above 20,000 feet).

Physiologic adaptation, although well characterized for various altitudes, should not be relied on at extremes of altitude. Nonetheless, as discussed in Chapter 4, physiologic adaptation has allowed people to reach the summit of Mount Everest *without supplemental oxygen.*

Clinical Problem 1.1. Two men first climbed the summit of Mount Everest without supplemental oxygen in 1978, and others have done so since. What major physiologic adaptation do you suppose makes such a climb possible?

One final point should be emphasized when discussing environmental pressures. The average *airway pressure* in the lungs will always equal the ambient or barometric pressure. (This is true during spontaneous breathing, i.e., without mechanical assistance. With mechanical ventilation, the average airway pressure will be slightly higher than ambient, the difference depending on the amount of positive pressure being delivered by the ventilator.)

When supplemental oxygen is breathed, the extra oxygen displaces nitrogen from the body's tissues. The amount of nitrogen displaced depends on the FIO_2 and how long the supplemental oxygen has been inhaled; but at any FIO_2, the total gaseous pressure remains atmospheric (i.e., equal to barometric pressure). Oxygen pressure merely replaces the nitrogen pressure. Breathing 100% oxygen over a sufficient period of time will totally denitrogenate the tissues, a fact that becomes important when considering alveolar PO_2 (Chapter 4).

Clinical Problem 1.2. What is the average airway pressure of a:

a. Denver resident?
b. New Orleans resident?
c. Climber in the Andes?
d. Climber on the summit of Mount Everest?
e. Subject breathing air in a hyperbaric chamber pressurized to 2 atm?

Clinical Problem 1.3. Denver's elevation is 1 mile (5,280 feet). Assuming barometric pressure changes linearly with altitude, what is the dry air PO_2 in Leadville, Colorado (altitude 10,200 feet), the highest incorporated city in the United States?

Clinical Problem 1.4. What is the total pressure of all gases in the lungs, apart from water vapor, under the following conditions:

a. P_B = 760 mm Hg, normal body temperature (37°C)?
b. P_B = 253 mm Hg, normal body temperature?
c. P_B = 760 mm Hg, body temperature 39°C? (Is it more or less than your answer for 1.4a?)

Clinical Problem 1.5. In general terms, what are the physiologic consequences during an airplane trip from the East Coast to California for someone who

a. Is healthy, with PaO_2 = 95 mm Hg?
b. Has mild chronic obstructive pulmonary disease (COPD) with PaO_2 75 mm Hg?
c. Has severe COPD with PaO_2 58 mm Hg?

Clinical Problem 1.6. You take a hot-air balloon ride from sea level to an altitude of 4000 feet. At this altitude, will the following values be higher, lower, or the same as they are at sea level?

a. FIO_2
b. Barometric pressure
c. PaO_2
d. Water vapor pressure in your lungs
e. Your average airway pressure
f. The sum of all the individual partial pressures (including water vapor pressure) in your alveoli

ANSWERS TO CLINICAL PROBLEMS

1.1. The alveolar gas equation, introduced in the next chapter, shows that alveolar PO_2 is directly related to the inspired oxygen pressure and inversely related to the $PaCO_2$. The inspired oxygen pressure is fixed by the FIO_2 and barometric pressure. Mountain climbers adapt at altitude principally by lowering $PaCO_2$, thereby raising their alveolar (and arterial) PO_2.

1.2. The average airway pressure in any location equals the barometric pressure at that location (Fig. 1.2). Although the barometric pressure fluctuates slightly during the day, knowledge of the average barometric pressure at a particular altitude is sufficient for blood gas interpretation purposes. In Denver, average airway pressure is 640 mm Hg; in New Orleans (sea level), it is 760 mm Hg. For the Andes, the answer, of course, depends on the specific altitude, but 380 mm Hg is the barometric pressure (and hence the airway pressure) at some of the peaks. On the summit of Mount Everest, the barometric pressure has been measured at 253 mm Hg. Finally, in a hyperbaric chamber, the ambient pressure is determined by the chamber. At 2 atm, the ambient pressure is

$$2 \times 760 \text{ mm Hg} = 1520 \text{ mm Hg}$$

which is also the average airway pressure of anyone in the chamber.

1.3. You are not expected to know the barometric pressure in Leadville, Colorado. However, from Figure 1.2 you can determine that P_B falls about 120 mm Hg per mile of altitude. Since Leadville is almost 2 miles high, the P_B is about 520 mm Hg. Since FIO_2 is 0.21, the dry air PO_2 in Leadville is approximately 109 mm Hg (compared to 160 mm Hg at sea level).

1.4.

a. Airway pressure = barometric pressure = 760 mm Hg. Water vapor pressure at 37°C = 47 mm Hg, which is subtracted to give the total gas pressure of 713 mm Hg (the sum of the partial pressures of oxygen, nitrogen, and carbon dioxide in the lungs at sea level).
b. By the same reasoning as in 1.4a, the total dry gas pressure is (253 − 47) mm Hg, or 206 mm Hg.
c. A febrile patient has a higher than normal water vapor pressure. At 39°C, water vapor pressure is about 52.4 mm Hg, 5.4 mm Hg higher than normal; subtracting this value from the barometric pressure of 760 mm Hg gives a dry gas pressure of about 707.6 mm Hg. (You are not expected to know the water vapor pressure at 39°C; a satisfactory answer to this question is "slightly lower than 713"). With most

changes in body temperature, the change in dry gas pressure (sum of oxygen, nitrogen, and carbon dioxide pressures) is trivial; for this reason, water vapor pressure, for clinical purposes, is usually assumed to equal 47 mm Hg.

1.5. In all three examples, the arterial PO_2 can be expected to fall because of the drop in P_B, although the fall will be lessened by mild hyperventilation. Regardless of how high the plane flies, the fall in P_B is limited to a cabin pressure equal to about 7000 feet altitude, so the physiologic consequences for the healthy person are obviously insignificant. The drop in PaO_2 will be more significant for the patient with mild COPD, but it should pose no clinical problem if resting PaO_2 at sea level is 75 mm Hg. Patients with severe lung impairment, on the other hand, must be cautioned about airplane travel; a patient with PaO_2 in the 50s should either not fly or receive supplemental oxygen en route, which can be provided by the airlines.

1.6.

a. Same.
b. Lower.
c. Lower; there will be some hyperventilation, but not enough to compensate for the fall in PaO_2 from the lower barometric pressure.
d. Same.
e. Lower.
f. Lower; this is essentially the same question as 1.6e.

CHAPTER

2

Three Physiologic Processes, Four Equations

THREE PHYSIOLOGIC PROCESSES

A student's first clinical exposure to arterial blood gases may be in the context of a senior physician saying "Let's check her PO_2" or asking "What's his PCO_2?" Certainly, a basic reason for the blood gas test is to find out a patient's PaO_2, $PaCO_2$, or pH. But why do we want these values? What do they really tell us? In conjunction with other laboratory and clinical information, pH, PaO_2, and $PaCO_2$ help assess three vital physiologic processes:

- Alveolar ventilation
- Oxygenation
- Acid–base balance

The only reason to obtain any blood gas measurement is to assess alveolar ventilation, oxygenation, and/or acid–base balance. That is really what interpreting blood gases is all about. If there were a quicker and easier way to obtain this assessment, the arterial blood gas test would become obsolete.

Even if noninvasive methods became widely available for measuring pH, $PaCO_2$, and PaO_2 (as they have for SaO_2; see Chapter 6), there would still be a need for clinical interpretation. Methodology for laboratory tests changes frequently; the physiology of alveolar ventilation, oxygenation, and acid–base balance is determined by nature and does not vary. For clinical purposes, the particular lab method that produces the data is not as important as understanding and using the information to benefit the patient.

FOUR IMPORTANT EQUATIONS

Four basic equations are necessary for both understanding and interpreting arterial blood gases:

	EQUATION	PHYSIOLOGIC PROCESS ASSESSED
1.	PCO_2	Alveolar ventilation
2.	Alveolar gas	Oxygenation
3.	Oxygen content	Oxygenation
4.	Henderson–Hasselbalch	Acid–base balance

These equations are clinically useful not so much for the numbers they generate as for their qualitative relationships. It is not important that you memorize these equations, now or ever. It *is* important that you learn the relationships among the variables they contain. As you read through this book and work on the problems, each equation and its clinical utility will become second nature to you. (Symbols used in these equations and elsewhere throughout the text are defined in Appendix C.)

1. PCO_2 equation

The PCO_2 equation puts into physiologic perspective one of the most common of all clinical observations: a patient's respiratory rate and breathing effort. This equation states that alveolar PCO_2 ($PaCO_2$) is directly proportional to the amount of CO_2 produced by metabolism and delivered to the lungs ($\dot{V}CO_2$), and inversely proportional to the alveolar ventilation ($\dot{V}A$). Because $PaCO_2$ can be assumed to equal $PaCO_2$, this equation can be stated as follows:

$$PaCO_2 = \frac{\dot{V}CO_2 \times 0.863}{\dot{V}A}$$

where

$PaCO_2$ = arterial PCO2 (mm Hg)
$\dot{V}CO_2$ = the amount of CO_2 produced by metabolism and delivered to the lungs (mL CO_2/min at STPD)
0.863 = a constant that equates dissimilar units for $\dot{V}CO_2$ (mL CO_2/min measured at STPD) and $\dot{V}A$ (L/min measured at BTPS) to $PaCO_2$ (mm Hg)
$\dot{V}A$ = alveolar ventilation (L/min at BTPS) = $\dot{V}E - \dot{V}D$, where
$\dot{V}E$ = minute or total ventilation (L/min) = respiratory rate × tidal volume
$\dot{V}D$ = dead space ventilation (L/min) = respiratory rate × dead space volume

Clinical Problem 2.1. If CO_2 production stays the same and alveolar ventilation increases, $PaCO_2$ will

a. Rise
b. Fall
c. Stay the same

Clinical Problem 2.2. If alveolar ventilation stays the same and CO_2 production increases, $PaCO_2$ will

a. Rise
b. Fall
c. Stay the same

Clinical Problem 2.3. A woman running on a treadmill doubles her respiratory rate, heart rate, level of CO_2 production, and minute and alveolar ventilation. If her baseline $PaCO_2$ is 40 mm Hg, her $PaCO_2$ during exercise is

a. 20 mm Hg
b. 30 mm Hg
c. 40 mm Hg
d. Impossible to determine from information provided

Clinical Problem 2.4. A patient with severe emphysema has an FEV-1 second of 0.5 L (25% of predicted). His resting $PaCO_2$ is 45 mm Hg. What will happen to his $PaCO_2$ when he exercises if his minute and dead space ventilation do not increase?

a. Will increase along with increase in $\dot{V}CO_2$
b. Will remain unchanged
c. Will decrease as a result of exertional hyperventilation
d. Change will depend on oxygen consumption

2. Alveolar gas equation

The alveolar gas equation is essential to understanding any PaO_2 value and in assessing if the lungs are properly transferring oxygen to the blood. Is a PaO_2 of 28 mm Hg abnormal? How about 50 mm Hg? 95 mm Hg? To understand any PaO_2 value one also has to know the $PaCO_2$, FIO_2 (fraction of inspired oxygen), and barometric pressure, all components of the alveolar gas equation:

$$PAO_2 = PIO_2 - 1.2(PaCO_2)^*$$

where

PAO_2 = mean alveolar PO_2 (mm Hg)
PIO_2 = partial pressure of inspired (tracheal) O_2 (mm Hg) = $FIO_2\ (P_B - P_{H_2O})$,

where

FIO_2 = fraction of inspired oxygen (0.*xx*)
P_B = barometric pressure (mm Hg)
P_{H_2O} = water vapor pressure (mm Hg)
$PaCO_2$ = arterial PCO_2 (mm Hg)

Clinical Problem 2.5. If PIO_2 stays the same and $PaCO_2$ increases, alveolar PO_2 will

a. Increase
b. Decrease
c. Remain the same

Clinical Problem 2.6. If $PaCO_2$ stays the same and FIO_2 increases, alveolar PO_2 will

a. Increase
b. Decrease
c. Remain the same

---

*The equation presented here is widely used for clinical purposes. It is an abbreviation of the formally derived alveolar gas equation:

$$PAO_2 = PIO_2 - (PACO_2) \times [FIO_2 + \frac{(1 - FIO_2)}{R}]$$

As with the PCO_2 equation, PAO_2 is calculated assuming that $PaCO_2 = PACO_2$.

Clinical Problem 2.7. If both sea level barometric pressure and $PaCO_2$ fall by half, alveolar PO_2 will
a. Increase
b. Decrease
c. Remain the same

Clinical Problem 2.8. If PAO_2 increases above normal, PaO_2
a. Increases if the lungs are normal
b. Increases only if the lungs are normal and the patient is hyperventilating (has reduced $PaCO_2$)
c. Always increases

Clinical Problem 2.9. If PAO_2 decreases, PaO_2
a. Always decreases
b. Decreases only if the lungs are abnormal
c. Decreases only if the lungs are abnormal and the patient is hypoventilating (has elevated $PaCO_2$)

Clinical Problem 2.10. If increasing altitude is the only changing variable, PAO_2 will
a. Increase
b. Decrease
c. Remain the same

Chapter 4 will discuss the relationship of PAO_2 to PaO_2 and clinical application of the "A–a O_2 difference."

3. Oxygen content equation

Oxygen is a gas and exerts a pressure, of course; but oxygen also has content. The oxygen content in the blood is recorded as CaO_2 (mL O_2/dL blood). CaO_2 is calculated by the oxygen content equation:

$$CaO_2 = \text{amount of } O_2 \text{ bound to hemoglobin} + \text{amount of } O_2 \text{ dissolved in plasma} = (SaO_2 \times Hb \times 1.34) + 0.003(PaO_2)$$

where

CaO_2 = mL O_2/dL arterial blood
SaO_2 = percent saturation of arterial hemoglobin with oxygen, expressed as decimal fraction (e.g., 0.98)
Hb = hemoglobin content (g/dL blood)
1.34 = O_2-binding capacity of hemoglobin (mL O_2/g Hb)
0.003 = solubility constant for dissolved O_2 in plasma = 0.003 mL O_2/dL/mm Hg PaO_2

Chapter 5 will explore in greater detail the difference between PaO_2 (oxygen pressure) and CaO_2 (oxygen content). Keep in mind that the body requires some quantity of oxygen molecules delivered each minute, a need that is met by cardiac output and arterial oxygen content. (The arterial oxygen content times the cardiac output is the arterial oxygen delivery, in mL O_2/min.)

Clinical Problem 2.11. If hemoglobin content decreases by 25%, CaO_2 will fall by

a. A lower percentage
b. A higher percentage
c. Approximately the same percentage

Clinical Problem 2.12. If SaO_2 falls by 25%, CaO_2 will fall by

a. Approximately the same percentage
b. A lower percentage
c. A higher percentage

Clinical Problem 2.13. A doubling of PaO_2 from 50 to 100 mm Hg, with no change in hemoglobin content, will

a. Double the CaO_2
b. Increase CaO_2 by more than 25%
c. Increase CaO_2 by less than 25%

Clinical Problem 2.14. If normal PaO_2 and oxygen contents are, respectively, 100 mm Hg and 20 mL O_2/dL, approximately what percent of oxygen content is contributed by the dissolved fraction of oxygen?

a. 1.5%
b. 3.0%
c. 4.5%

Clinical Problem 2.15. If a patient's PaO_2 is 100 mm Hg but, because of anemia, CaO_2 (arterial oxygen content) is only 10 mL O_2/dL, what percentage of CaO_2 is contributed by the dissolved fraction of oxygen?

a. 1.5%
b. 3.0%
c. 4.5%

4. The Henderson–Hasselbalch equation

The Henderson–Hasselbalch (H–H) equation is perhaps the most familiar of the four equations important for basic blood gas interpretation. The H–H equation relates pH to components of the bicarbonate buffer system, the largest buffer system in the extracellular fluid. Any blood acid–base disturbance is instantaneously reflected in one or both of its buffer components (HCO_3^- and $PaCO_2$); their ratio at any one time determines the blood's acidity, as defined by pH in the H–H equation.

$$pH = pK + \log \frac{HCO_3^-}{0.03(PaCO_2)}$$

where

pH = the negative logarithm of hydrogen ion concentration
pK = 6.1, the negative logarithm of the dissociation constant for car bonic acid
HCO_3^- = the concentration of bicarbonate (mEq/L)
$PaCO_2$ = partial pressure of CO_2 in arterial blood (mm Hg)
0.03 = solubility coefficient for PCO_2 in plasma (mEq/L/mm Hg)

Because the H–H equation incorporates a logarithm, shortened versions have been promulgated for rapid calculation of $[H^+]$ and HCO_3^- (see Chapter 7); however, as with the other three equations, calculations are not as important as understanding the relationship among the variables.

Clinical Problem 2.16. If HCO_3^- and $PaCO_2$ double from their normal baseline values, pH will

a. Stay the same
b. Double
c. Depend on the change in pK of the buffer system

Clinical Problem 2.17. If HCO_3^- falls by half and $PaCO_2$ remains the same, pH will

a. Stay the same
b. Increase
c. Decrease

Clinical Problem 2.18. A pH of 7.40 means

a. HCO_3^- is normal
b. $PaCO_2$ is normal
c. The ratio of HCO_3^- to $PaCO_2$ is normal

Clinical Problem 2.19. If $PaCO_2$ increases from 40 to 60 mm Hg, the H–H equation predicts

a. pH will fall
b. Bicarbonate will fall
c. Bicarbonate will rise
d. Nothing, since change in a single H–H variable cannot predict change in the other two

There are many other equations and formulas one can explore in a discussion of blood gas interpretation. The point is not to belabor equations but to emphasize qualitative relationships among key variables. If you learn well the relationships expressed in these four equations you will seldom, if ever, have to do any calculations.

Clinical Problem 2.20. If CO_2 production, PIO_2, and HCO_3^- remain constant, then as alveolar ventilation decreases ________________ and ________________ will also decrease.

Clinical Problem 2.21. If both PIO_2 and HCO_3^- remain constant, then as $PaCO_2$ increases, ______________ and ________________ will decrease.

Clinical Problem 2.22. The relationship of PaO_2 to CaO_2 has not been presented but you may already know it. How would you describe this relationship: Linear? Curvilinear? Reciprocal?

____

____

Clinical Problem 2.23. Changes in which of the following will not affect the PAO_2? (**Hint:** stick to the basic equations.)

a. $PaCO_2$
b. SaO_2
c. Hemoglobin content
d. HCO_3^-
e. Altitude
f. Barometric pressure
g. FIO_2
h. Patient's age

Write the four equations just presented in the spaces provided below; then check your responses by referring to the previous pages. Remember: **Correct expression of the relationships is more important than memorizing constants or doing the actual calculations.** Please make sure you know the correct relationships for each equation before proceeding to Chapter 3.

PCO_2 equation:

$PaCO_2$ =

Alveolar gas equation:

PAO_2 =

Oxygen content equation:

CaO_2 =

Henderson–Hasselbalch equation:

pH =

ANSWERS TO CLINICAL PROBLEMS

The questions in this chapter are designed to orient you to changes in relationships rather than to doing calculations. All the questions can be answered with reference to one or more of the four equations just presented.

2.1. b. The $PaCO_2$ equation states that $PaCO_2$ is directly related to CO_2 production and inversely related to alveolar ventilation. Hence if CO_2 production stays the same and alveolar ventilation increases, $PaCO_2$ has to fall.

2.2. a. Use the same reasoning as in 2.1: If alveolar ventilation stays the same and CO_2 production increases, $PaCO_2$ will rise.

2.3. c. In this problem, the subject doubles her rate of CO_2 production and alveolar ventilation. Since both values double, her exercise $PaCO_2$ should remain unchanged at 40 mm Hg.

2.4. a. This problem is qualitatively similar to Clinical Problem 2.2. By definition, fixed minute and dead space ventilation means that alveolar ventilation is unchanged. Since CO_2 production increases with exercise and alveolar ventilation (in this case) remains unchanged, $PaCO_2$ should increase. Note that oxygen consumption is not a variable in the $PaCO_2$ equation.

2.5. b. The alveolar gas equation states that PAO_2 goes up with increases in PIO_2 and down with increases in $PaCO_2$. Hence if PIO_2 remains the same and $PaCO_2$ increases, alveolar PO_2 will decrease.

2.6. a. If $PaCO_2$ stays the same and FIO_2 increases, alveolar PO_2 will increase.

2.7. b. In this example, sea level barometric pressure (760 mm Hg) and baseline $PaCO_2$ (40 mm Hg) each fall by half. A fall in P_B will lower, whereas a fall in $PaCO_2$ will raise, the alveolar PO_2. A brief calculation shows that, percentage-wise, reducing $PaCO_2$ cannot compensate for decreases in barometric pressure. In this example PAO_2 will decrease.

2.8. a. When PAO_2 increases, PaO_2 will also increase if the lungs are normal. This occurs whether or not the person with normal lungs hyperventilates; hence answer b is incorrect. If the lungs are diseased, PaO_2 may not go up with increases in PAO_2; hence answer c is incorrect.

2.9. a. Since oxygen enters the blood by passive diffusion, PAO_2 defines the upper limit of PaO_2. Any decrease of PAO_2 will be reflected in a decrease of PaO_2. Note that the opposite is not true, since the lower limit of PaO_2 is determined by the state of the lungs (ventilation–perfusion relationships).

2.10. b. Increasing altitude is associated with decreasing barometric pressure, so the PAO_2 will decrease.

2.11. c. If hemoglobin content decreases by 25%, CaO_2 will fall by approximately the same percentage ("approximately" because the dissolved O_2 fraction, which accounts for very little of the oxygen content, will not change as hemoglobin falls).

2.12. a. Same reasoning as in 2.11.

2.13. c. Doubling PaO_2 from 50 to 100 mm Hg, with no change in hemoglobin content, will change the CaO_2 according to the change in the variables in the O_2 content equation. PaO_2 values of 50 and 100 mm Hg represent an oxygen saturation of about 85 and 98%, respectively. Hence CaO_2 will increase by less than 25%.

2.14. a. Since dissolved fraction = 0.003 mL O_2/dL × PaO_2, the amount of dissolved oxygen is 0.3 mL/dL. This comes to 1.5% of the total.

2.15. b. Since the PaO_2 is the same as in problem 2.13, the dissolved component is 0.3 mL O_2/dL. However, since the oxygen content is only 10 mL O_2/dL, half that in problem 2.13, the percentage contributed by dissolved oxygen is double, or 3%.

2.16. a. The H–H equation states that pH is directly related to the ratio of HCO_3^- over $PaCO_2$. Hence if HCO_3^- and $PaCO_2$ double from their normal baseline value, their ratio and the resulting pH will stay the same.

2.17. c. If HCO_3^- falls by half and $PaCO_2$ remains the same, pH will decrease.

2.18. c. A pH of 7.40 means only that the ratio of HCO_3^- to $PaCO_2$ is normal.

2.19. d. The H–H equation per se predicts nothing from a change in only one variable. Although acute CO_2 retention is manifested by a reduced pH and slight elevation of HCO_3^-, these changes are not predicted by the equation.

2.20. Based on the equations presented in this chapter, if CO_2 production, PIO_2, and HCO_3^- remain constant, then, as alveolar ventilation decreases, pH and PAO_2 will also decrease.

2.21. If PIO_2 and HCO_3^- remain constant, then, as $PaCO_2$ increases, pH and PAO_2 will decrease.

2.22. The relation of PaO_2 to CaO_2 is the same as the relation of PaO_2 to SaO_2, i.e., a sigmoid-shaped curve.

2.23. Changes in the following parameters will not affect the PAO_2: SaO_2, hemoglobin content, HCO_3^-, and patient's age. $PaCO_2$, barometric pressure, altitude (through its effect on barometric pressure), and FIO_2 are variables in the alveolar gas equation and so will affect the PAO_2.

CHAPTER

3

$PaCO_2$ and Alveolar Ventilation

HIGH AND LOW $PaCO_2$

As with any single laboratory value, $PaCO_2$ can be either high or low. Because normal $PaCO_2$ is 35–45 mm Hg, a $PaCO_2 > 45$ mm Hg is "high" and < 35 mm Hg is "low." Of course, proper interpretation of $PaCO_2$ is somewhat more sophisticated (or you wouldn't be reading this book!).

In discussing $PaCO_2$ there should be some agreement on terminology. *Hypercapnia* and *hypocapnia* are the terms for high and low $PaCO_2$, respectively. Note that the opposite prefix denotes the respective state of alveolar ventilation.

$PaCO_2$, mm Hg	CONDITION IN BLOOD	STATE OF ALVEOLAR VENTILATION
> 45	Hypercapnia	Hypoventilation
35–45	Eucapnia	Normal ventilation
< 35	Hypocapnia	Hyperventilation

The reason that hypercapnia reflects a state of hypoventilation is shown by the $PaCO_2$ equation, first introduced in Chapter 2:

$$PaCO_2 = \frac{\dot{V}CO_2 \text{ (mL/min)} \times 0.863}{\dot{V}A \text{ (L/min)}}$$

Alveolar ventilation ($\dot{V}A$) is the total amount of air breathed in per minute ($\dot{V}E$; expired or minute ventilation) minus the air that goes to all the dead space per minute ($\dot{V}D$).

$$\dot{V}A = \dot{V}E - \dot{V}D$$

where

$\dot{V}E$ = respiratory rate × tidal volume
$\dot{V}D$ = respiratory rate × dead space volume

Figure 3.1 shows the separation of dead space and alveolar space and their respective ventilations. Schematics like Figure 3.1, often reproduced in textbooks, suggest the volumes are fixed, although they are not. The dead space volume (150 mL in this case) represents nonventilating airways (the upper airway, bronchi, and bronchioles) and thus reflects airways that don't (and can never) take part in actual gas exchange. But alveoli, which are gas exchanging airways, can be converted into dead space when they are unperfused or underperfused, as commonly happens in many lung diseases.

Thus there are really two dead space volumes, commonly referred to as anatomic and physiologic. Anatomic dead space includes all the airways that can never take part in gas exchange, i.e., all airways down to the alveolar level. Physiologic dead space includes all the anatomic dead space plus the alveolar spaces that receive air but, because of perfusion irregularities, do not allow some or all of the contained air to participate in gas exchange.

Since all alveoli normally take part in gas exchange the distinction between the two dead spaces is not important in the healthy individual. The normal ratio of physiologic (or total) dead space to tidal volume (VD/VT) is about one-third, or 167 mL, for a tidal volume of 500 mL.

In pulmonary disease, however, the VD/VT ratio can greatly increase, as a result of a severe ventilation–perfusion imbalance. For example, in a patient with severe emphysema, 300 mL, or 60% of a tidal volume of 500 mL, could go to satisfy the dead space. Here the extra dead space comes about largely because of

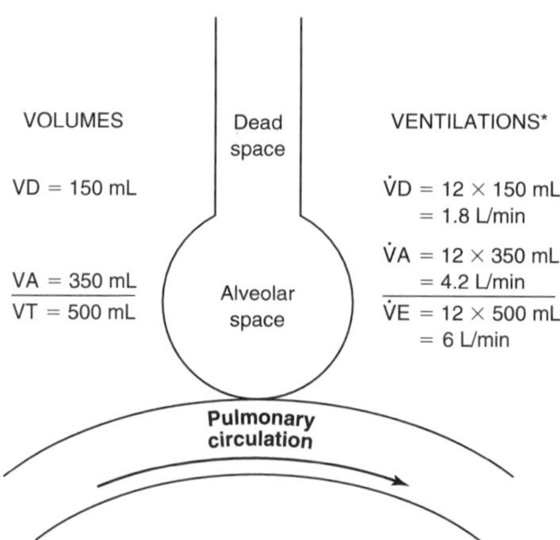

Figure 3.1. The difference between lung volumes and ventilations. *Respiratory rate = 12/min. See text for discussion.

air that enters alveoli but exchanges gases ineffectively or not at all. This "nonexchanging" air in the alveolar spaces is just as "wasted" as air entering the trachea and bronchi. Because of the large amount of wasted ventilation, the patient would likely manifest dyspnea owing to the increased work of breathing.

The dead space in the $PaCO_2$ equation is the physiologic or total dead space. The symbol in the denominator, $\dot{V}D$, thus represents the amount of air entering the physiologic dead space per minute, i.e., all the air that does not take part in gas exchange.

Clinical Problem 3.1. What are the dead space volume and $\dot{V}D$ if the tidal volume is 500 mL, respiratory rate is 12/min, and $\dot{V}A = 3$ L/min?

Clinical Problem 3.2. Does the volume calculated in Clinical Problem 3.1 represent the anatomic or physiologic dead space?

From the $PaCO_2$ equation it is evident that hypoventilation resulting in elevated $PaCO_2$ is really "hypo-alveolar-ventilation relative to CO_2 production." Similarly, hyperventilation leading to low $PaCO_2$ is really "hyper-alveolar-ventilation relative to CO_2 production." By convention, the terms *alveolar* and *relative to CO_2 production* are omitted when characterizing the state of ventilation as it relates to $PaCO_2$.

Notice that the only number needed for determining the patient's state of alveolar ventilation is the $PaCO_2$. We do not need to know the actual amount of alveolar ventilation or CO_2 production (they are not routine measurements and are never reported with routine blood gas values).

Clinically, we need to know only if a patient's $\dot{V}A$ is adequate for $\dot{V}CO_2$; if it is, then $PaCO_2$ will be in the normal range (35–45 mm Hg). Conversely, a normal $PaCO_2$ means only that alveolar ventilation is adequate for the patient's level of CO_2 production at the moment $PaCO_2$ was measured.

In summary, the terms *hypoventilation* and *hyperventilation* refer only to high or low $PaCO_2$, respectively. For reasons that will be discussed subsequently, these terms should not be used to characterize any patient's rate or depth of respirations or the work of breathing.

Clinical Problem 3.3. What is the $PaCO_2$ of a patient with respiratory rate = 24/min, tidal volume = 300 mL, dead space volume = 150 mL, and CO_2 production = 300 mL/min? The patient shows some evidence of respiratory distress.

Clinical Problem 3.4. Is the patient described in Clinical Problem 3.3 hyperventilating, hypoventilating, or normally ventilating?

Clinical Problem 3.5. What is the $PaCO_2$ of a patient with respiratory rate = 10/min, tidal volume = 600 mL, dead space volume = 150 mL, and CO_2 production = 200 mL/min? The patient shows some evidence of respiratory distress.

Clinical Problem 3.6. Is the patient described in Clinical Problem 3.5 hyperventilating, hypoventilating or normally ventilating?

Clinical Problem 3.7. Which of the following patients can be said to be hyperventilating?

a. A 50-year-old man with respiratory rate = 30/min who uses accessory muscles of breathing
b. A comatose 29-year-old woman with respiratory rate = 8/min and $PaCO_2$ = 28 mm Hg
c. A 65-year-old man with tidal volume = 400 mL and respiratory rate = 22/min

Examine the following statement and decide whether it is true or false before reading further:

The only physiologic reason for elevated $PaCO_2$ is a level of alveolar ventilation inadequate for the amount of CO_2 produced and delivered to the lungs.

Since $PaCO_2$ equals CO_2 production over alveolar ventilation—and nothing else—this is a true statement. Note the emphasis on inadequate alveolar ventilation as opposed to excess CO_2 production. This is because excess CO_2 production is not a problem for the normal respiratory system.

If excess CO_2 production were to cause hypercapnia, you would expect to see it during exercise, when CO_2 production is greatly augmented. During submaximal exercise (below the point of anaerobic threshold) $\dot{V}CO_2$ goes up owing to exercising muscles, but $PaCO_2$ stays in the normal range. Why? Because $\dot{V}A$ rises proportionally to the rise in $\dot{V}CO_2$. With extremes of exercise (beyond the anaerobic threshold), $PaCO_2$ falls as compensation for the developing lactic acidosis. In a healthy individual undergoing strenuous exercise, when the highest levels of CO_2 production are reached, $PaCO_2$ may be reduced (normal hyperventilation) but it is never elevated.

At this point you should understand that the physiologic basis of all hypercapnia is alveolar ventilation inadequate for CO_2 production. With that understanding, you can now appreciate the clinical reasons for an elevated $PaCO_2$. Because $\dot{V}A = \dot{V}E - \dot{V}D$, any elevated $PaCO_2$ can be explained by one of the following situations:

a. *Inadequate $\dot{V}E$.* This may occur from central nervous system depression (e.g., drug overdose), respiratory muscle weakness or paralysis (e.g., polio, myasthenia gravis), or any other condition that limits rate or depth of breathing (e.g., massive obesity, severe pulmonary fibrosis).
b. *Too much of the $\dot{V}E$ goes to $\dot{V}D$.* This situation is common in severe chronic obstructive pulmonary disease (COPD), in which the architecture of the alveolar spaces is altered, so that alveoli are ventilated but unperfused or underperfused. The result is creation of physiologic dead space. Excess $\dot{V}D$ can also occur when breathing is rapid and shallow, sometimes seen in severe restrictive impairment (e.g., pulmonary fibrosis).
c. *Some combination of a and b.* This may occur, for example, in a patient with both severe COPD and muscle fatigue. The COPD gives an increase in $\dot{V}D$, and the fatigue makes it difficult for the patient to sustain an adequate minute ventilation.

ASSESSING ALVEOLAR VENTILATION AT THE BEDSIDE

An important clinical corollary of the $PaCO_2$ equation is that one cannot reliably assess the adequacy of alveolar ventilation, and hence $PaCO_2$, at the bedside. $\dot{V}E$ can easily be measured with a handheld spirometer (as tidal volume times respiratory rate), but there is no way to know the amount of $\dot{V}E$ going to dead space or the patient's rate of CO_2 production ($\dot{V}CO_2$). A common mistake is to assume that someone who is breathing fast, hard, and/or deep is always hyperventilating. Not so, of course.

CASE. *An intern is called to the hospital bedside of an elderly woman late at night. The patient was admitted to the hospital 3 days earlier for a problem unrelated to her heart or lungs. She is anxious and complains of shortness of breath. Her lung fields are clear to auscultation and vital signs are normal except for slight tachycardia and a respiratory rate of 30/min. A nurse comments that the patient "gets like this every night." The physician orders an antianxiety drug for what he describes as "hyperventilation and anxiety." About 30 minutes later, the patient's breathing slows considerably and she becomes cyanotic, whereupon she is transferred to the intensive care unit.*

What would you guess this patient's blood gas values were before she received the antianxiety drug?

a. $PaCO_2$ = 32 mm Hg, PaO_2 = 70 mm Hg
b. $PaCO_2$ = 43 mm Hg, PaO_2 = 80 mm Hg
c. $PaCO_2$ = 58 mm Hg, PaO_2 = 62 mm Hg

Although nothing in the PCO_2 equation directly relates respiratory rate or depth of breathing to $PaCO_2$, such observations are commonly (and mistakenly) used to assess a patient's $PaCO_2$. The error in this case was to assume the patient was hyperventilating (because she was breathing fast) and could tolerate the sedative; in fact she was hypoventilating and hypoxemic (answer c). She had undiagnosed COPD and chronic hypercapnia.

Hypercapnia represents a failure of some component of the respiratory system (comprising the central nervous system; thoracic cage, including the diaphragm; and lungs and airways) and, therefore, indicates a state of advanced organ system impairment. The potential causes are many and varied, ranging from stable COPD to acute pulmonary edema, from chronic opiate ingestion to severe interstitial lung disease. The clinical presentation is equally varied, from no distress to the need for emergency resuscitation.

In addition to advanced organ system impairment, there are three physiologic reasons why an elevated $PaCO_2$ is potentially dangerous.

- As $PaCO_2$ increases, PAO_2 and PaO_2 fall, unless inspired oxygen is supplemented (see Chapter 4).
- As $PaCO_2$ increases, pH falls, unless HCO_3^- also increases (see Chapter 7).
- The higher the $PaCO_2$, the less defended the patient is against any further decline in $\dot{V}A$.

This last point is illustrated by plotting $PaCO_2$ against alveolar ventilation (Fig. 3.2). The higher the $PaCO_2$ to begin with, the more it will rise for any given decrement in $\dot{V}A$. For example, when $\dot{V}CO_2$ is 200 mL/min, a decrease in $\dot{V}A$ of 1 L/min (as may occur from anesthesia, sedation, pneumonia, and other causes) will increase a patient's baseline $PaCO_2$ of 29 mm Hg to 34.5 mm Hg. The same 1 L/min decline in alveolar ventilation will raise a baseline PCO_2 of 60 mm Hg to 90 mm Hg.

Clinical Problem 3.8. Given a $\dot{V}CO_2$ of 300 mL/min, state the change in $PaCO_2$ that will result from a 1 L/min decrease in $\dot{V}A$ when baseline $PaCO_2$ is:

a. 30 mm Hg
b. 40 mm Hg
c. 50 mm Hg

Clinical Problem 3.9. Given a fixed alveolar ventilation of 4 L/min, calculate the $PaCO_2$ for each of the following rates of CO_2 production.

a. 200 mL/min
b. 300 mL/min
c. 400 mL/min

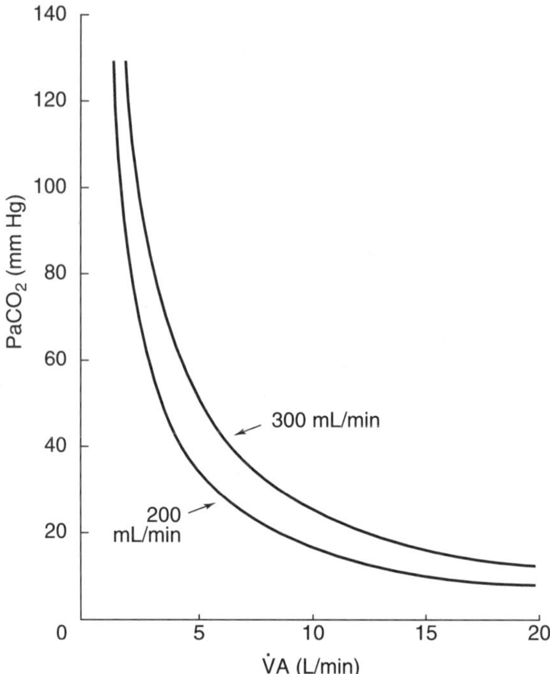

Figure 3.2. $PaCO_2$ vs. alveolar ventilation ($\dot{V}A$) for carbon dioxide production rates of 200 and 300 mL/min. A decrease in alveolar ventilation in the hypercapnic patient results in a greater rise in $PaCO_2$ than the same $\dot{V}A$ change when $PaCO_2$ is low or normal. Furthermore, an increase in carbon dioxide production when $\dot{V}A$ is fixed results in an increase in $PaCO_2$.

> **Clinical Problem 3.10.** A severely emphysematous patient exercises on a treadmill at 3 mph. His rate of CO_2 production increases by 50%, but he is unable to augment alveolar ventilation. If his resting $PaCO_2$ is 40 mm Hg and resting $\dot{V}CO_2$ is 200 mL/min, what will his exercise $PaCO_2$ be?

NONINVASIVE MEASUREMENT OF PCO_2—CAPNOGRAPHY

Measurement of the end-tidal PCO_2 (or $PetCO_2$) is achieved noninvasively by analyzing the fraction of CO_2 in expired air. $PetCO_2$ can often substitute for $PaCO_2$ and thus obviate drawing an arterial blood sample. This is so because, in most clinical situations, $PetCO_2$ either closely approximates $PaCO_2$ or differs from $PaCO_2$ by some fairly constant amount.

The measurement of CO_2 in expired gas is called capnography. Capnography can be done on a continuous basis, using either an infrared analyzer or a mass spectrometer (Clark et al. 1992; Stock 1995; Wright 1992). Most intensive care units employ infrared capnography, since it is much cheaper to monitor a group of patients with this method than with a mass spectrometer.

Capnography is widely used in intubated patients, where it is easy to ensure a closed circuit and no sample contamination from room air. Capnography can also be done in spontaneously breathing patients with a special nasal cannula to capture the exhaled gas (Liu et al. 1992). Because it is often difficult to prevent room air contamination in spontaneously breathing patients, capnography is not widely used in this group. The remainder of this discussion is based on experience with intubated, mechanically-ventilated patients.

In ventilated patients, the sensor for exhaled carbon dioxide is placed in the ventilator tubing so that it can measure both inspired and expired air. $PetCO_2$ is continuously displayed on the bedside monitor. The curve registering $PetCO_2$ goes up and peaks or plateaus with expiration and returns to baseline (zero) with inspiration (Fig. 3.3). A bedside monitor can graphically display

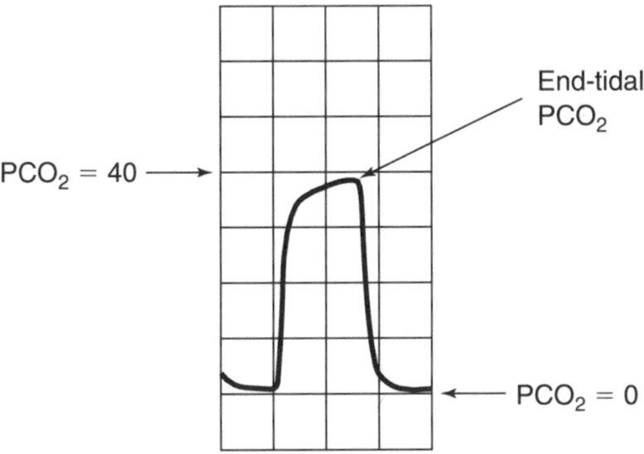

Figure 3.3. Single breath display of inhaled and exhaled CO_2. The inhaled PCO_2 is zero (the amount in inhaled air is negligible); the first part of exhaled air reflects air recently inhaled and also has a PCO_2 of zero. This is followed by air that is a mixture of alveolar and dead space gas, which contains increasing amounts of CO_2, until finally a peak or plateau is reached that, ideally, reflects air only from the alveoli. This peak or plateau is the end-tidal point, and its PCO_2 is the end-tidal PCO_2 ($PetCO_2$). In health, $PetCO_2$ is equal or close to the alveolar and arterial PCO_2; in this example, $PetCO_2$ = 38 mm Hg and $PaCO_2$ at that point = 40 mm Hg.

the breath-to-breath changes in CO_2 as well as the digital value of the end-tidal CO_2 as a percentage or as a pressure (Fig. 3.4).

Figure 3.3 shows a normal tracing of expired PCO_2 measured during a tidal volume breath; it was printed out to be placed in the patient's chart. The first part of the expired air is the same as the last part of the inspired air of the previous breath (it is dead space air from the upper airways and will contain almost no carbon dioxide).

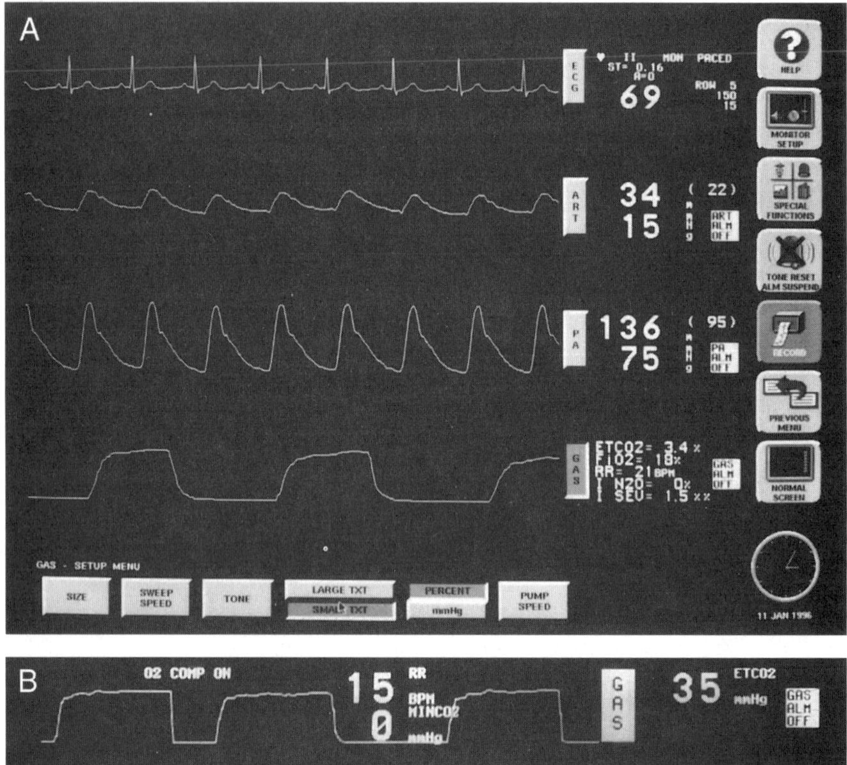

Figure 3.4. Monitor displays of end-tidal CO_2. **A,** The bottom tracing shows the sequence of breath-by-breath end-tidal CO_2 measurements ($ETCO_2$); also shown are the tracings of the ECG, pulmonary artery pressure, and systemic artery pressure. Here, $ETCO_2$ is registered as a percent (3.4%). If the dry gas pressure is 713 mm Hg, then $PetCO_2$ is 24.2 mm Hg. Courtesy Space Labs Medical, Redmond, WA. **B,** Breath-by-breath end-tidal CO_2 registered as a pressure reading. In this example, $PetCO_2$ = 35 mm Hg and the respiratory rate = 15/min.

Gradually, air from some of the alveoli begins to join this dead space air, and the PCO_2 rises. By the very end of exhalation, all the dead space air has left the lungs and the last few milliliters of air are from the alveoli only. The tracing shows that the $PetCO_2$ is approximately 38 mm Hg, which is very close to the $PaCO_2$.

$PetCO_2$ IN HEALTH AND DISEASE

In health, because carbon dioxide is never diffusion limited, alveolar PCO_2 ($PaCO_2$) is assumed equal to the end-capillary PCO_2, which in turn is equal to arterial PCO_2 ($PaCO_2$). Thus if you could sample alveolar PCO_2 you would have a proxy for $PaCO_2$. This in fact is possible because the last bit of air exhaled in each breath is the end-of-tidal-volume (end-tidal) air and comes from the alveoli. By sampling exhaled gas breath to breath, we can obtain a continuous display of the end-tidal PCO_2. This continuous reading should be equal or very close (within 1–2 mm Hg) to the alveolar and arterial PCO_2. To summarize, in health:

$$PetCO_2 \cong PaCO_2 \cong PaCO_2$$

In patients with lung disease and ventilation–perfusion (V–Q) imbalance, $PetCO_2$ will likely not be equal or close to the alveolar and arterial PCO_2. This is because of increased physiologic dead space common in states of V–Q imbalance. Increases in dead space come about when a group of alveoli are unperfused or underperfused, so that air reaching them becomes wholly or partly dead space air. Air in unperfused or underperfused alveoli keeps a low PCO_2, since little or no CO_2 is added to it (remember, inhaled air has almost zero CO_2). This concept is illustrated in Figure 3.5.

In Figure 3.5*A*, ventilation and perfusion in both lungs match so that the alveolar and arterial PCO_2 are the same (40 mm Hg). In Figure 3.5*B* one lung is unperfused, so that alveoli in that lung see only dead space air; as a result, the alveolar PCO_2 in that lung is same as in inhaled air, i.e., zero. The other lung remains well perfused, and gas exchange takes place normally. In fact, the blood maintains a $PaCO_2$ of 40 mm Hg because sufficient air is brought to the perfused lung to excrete the total metabolic CO_2 load.

In Figure 3.5*A*, the exhaled air reflects the alveolar PCO_2 and is equal or close to 40 mm Hg. In Figure 3.5*B*, the exhaled air also reflects the alveolar PCO_2 but includes all the dead space air from the unperfused lung; the mixture of dead space air and air from the perfused lung results in a low end-tidal PCO_2 (about 20 mm Hg).

All diseases manifested by a V–Q imbalance will have some regions of the

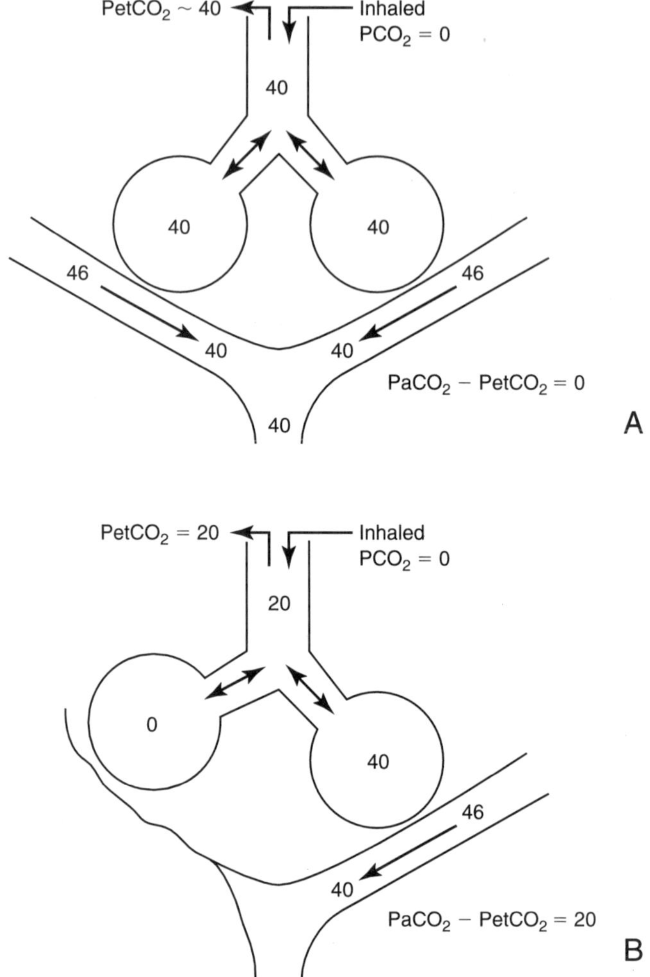

Figure 3.5. Normal and abnormal $PetCO_2$ (all values are in mm Hg). **A,** Normal ventilation–perfusion ratios. The arterial and alveolar PCO_2 values are equal; the last bit of alveolar air exhaled is the end-tidal PCO_2, which will have the same value as (or be close to) $PaCO_2$. **B,** Excess dead space ventilation will lower the $PetCO_2$, which commonly occurs whenever there is ventilation–perfusion imbalance. See text for discussion.

lung with high V–Q ratios; by definition, these regions will be relatively underperfused. The result will be an increased difference between $PetCO_2$ and $PaCO_2$.

Figure 3.6 is a breath-by-breath tracing of CO_2 from a patient with severe COPD. In this patient, the $PetCO_2$ averages approximately 50 mm Hg, but the

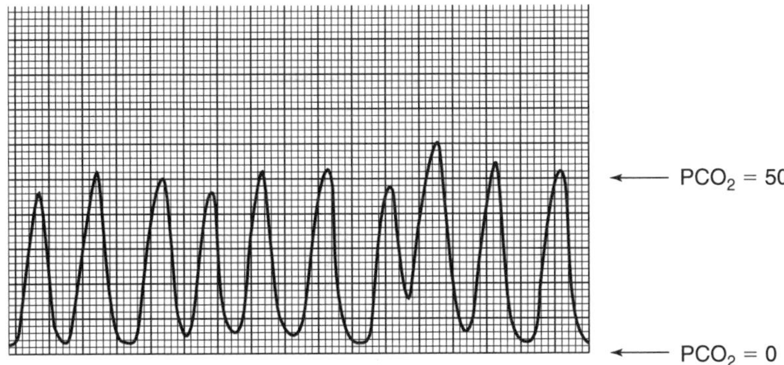

Figure 3.6. Continuous monitoring of end-tidal carbon dioxide ($PetCO_2$) in a patient with severe chronic obstructive pulmonary disease. The patient was tachypneic so that the breaths appear compressed. Note the slight variation in $PetCO_2$. The average $PetCO_2$ in this sequence of breaths is about 50 mm Hg. The patient's $PaCO_2$ measured at the same time was 74 mm Hg, for a $PaCO_2$-$PetCO_2$ of 24 mm Hg.

$PaCO_2$ is 74 mm Hg; the $PaCO_2$–$PetCO_2$ difference is 24 mm Hg. In this situation, the diseased alveoli do not empty evenly, and the end-tidal sample includes considerable dead space air.

There is no way to know how large the $PaCO_2$–$PetCO_2$ difference will be in a given patient or a given type of lung disease. And although 24 mm Hg is a relatively high difference between $PaCO_2$ and $PetCO_2$, a large difference does not obviate the usefulness of $PetCO_2$, as will be pointed out in the next section. Like any blood gas measurement, the result must be validated and interpreted in light of the full clinical picture.

PROPER USE OF END-TIDAL PCO_2

The principal advantages of capnography over intermittent measurement of arterial blood gases are (1) to obviate the need for blood sampling and (2) to allow for continuous reading of $PetCO_2$. Thus, to the extent that $PetCO_2$ can be used as a proxy for $PaCO_2$, it has obvious utility in the intensive care setting. When properly used, $PetCO_2$ (along with pulse oximetry) can often reduce arterial blood sampling and allow for safe patient monitoring.

There are two keys to using $PetCO_2$ properly: First, make a correlation with $PaCO_2$; and second, know the pitfalls that can affect interpretation of $PetCO_2$.

Correlate PetCO2 with $PaCO_2$

A sizable $PaCO_2$–$PetCO_2$ difference does not obviate the value of the $PetCO_2$ for physiologic monitoring. A rise in $PetCO_2$ still indicates a rise in $PaCO_2$, but one cannot equate the numerical value of $PetCO_2$ with $PaCO_2$. Therefore, for physiologic monitoring, at least one or two comparisons should be made between $PetCO_2$ and $PaCO_2$ before following $PetCO_2$. Once the difference between the two values is established, *and providing the patient remains clinically stable,* the $PetCO_2$ can be followed in lieu of the $PaCO_2$.

Below are some data from a stable 38-year-old man who is receiving mechanical ventilation. Assuming there is no major change in his clinical condition, how could you use $PetCO_2$ in weaning him from the ventilator?

ARTERIAL BLOOD GASES		$PetCO_2$
FIO_2	.40	
pH	7.41	
$PaCO_2$	56 mm Hg	35–40 mm Hg
PaO_2	70 mm Hg	
SaO_2	93%	
HCO_3^-	36mEq/L	

His $PetCO_2$ is 16–21 mm Hg lower than the arterial PCO_2. If he is stable, this difference can be added to the $PetCO_2$ during weaning to determine $PaCO_2$ at any time (± a few mm Hg). If the patient remains clinically stable, one should not have to obtain an arterial sample to measure $PaCO_2$. Of course, other parameters should also be followed, such as pulse oximetry and respiratory rate.

Know the pitfalls that can affect interpretation of $PetCO_2$

There are several potential pitfalls when interpreting the $PetCO_2$; but in the aggregate, they are not common and should not dissuade one from using $PetCO_2$ as a proxy for $PaCO_2$ in intubated patients. Although $PetCO_2$ is not as widely used as pulse oximetry and is, therefore, a less familiar measurement, properly used it can be a valuable monitoring aid. Potential pitfalls include the following.

1. With cardiac arrest, shock, or any other state of low pulmonary blood flow, $PetCO_2$ may be significantly and variably lower than $PaCO_2$, too much to use as a proxy for $PaCO_2$. In such conditions, it is best to measure $PaCO_2$ directly. Interestingly, however, changes in $PetCO_2$ can be used as a guide to changes in cardiac output (see below).
2. $PetCO_2$ may be higher than $PaCO_2$. Although this has been reported, it is not common (Moorthy et al. 1984; Stock 1995). It may occur transiently, for example, if a high inspired O_2 concentration displaces CO_2 from hemoglobin or if there is a sudden surge in CO_2 production. Because ultimately exhaled air must include some air recently inhaled (anatomic dead space air with zero CO_2), the reversal of gradient should be transient. The most common cause for reversal of gradient is probably when $PaCO_2$ and $PetCO_2$ are not measured at exactly the same time. Another potential cause is the inherent variation of laboratory measurements, so that if each is accurate within a few mm Hg, on occasion $PetCO_2$ may be higher. In any case, even when $PetCO_2$ is higher than $PaCO_2$, the difference is generally small ($<$ 5 mm Hg) and $PetCO_2$ can still be used to trend the $PaCO_2$, providing the patient is clinically stable. *Clinically stable* means no large changes in blood pressure, minute ventilation, temperature, or degree of physical activity (agitation, seizures, etc.) Within this framework, clinicians in the ICU know whether a patient is stable or not.
3. Another pitfall is not making a fresh correlation with $PaCO_2$ when there has been a significant clinical change. Sometimes $PetCO_2$ is followed for a prolonged period without blood gas correlation. Changes in the patient's metabolic condition, minute ventilation, and cardiopulmonary status can all affect the difference between end-tidal and arterial PCO_2. When there has been significant clinical or biochemical change, one should again make a correlation between $PetCO_2$ and $PaCO_2$.

CLINICAL USES OF $PetCO_2$

There is a large and growing literature on use of $PetCO_2$ in clinical medicine (Clark et al. 1992; Stock 1995; Wright 1992). Remember: Because $PetCO_2$ can be measured continuously, changes in ventilation that might be missed with intermittent blood gas monitoring are easily spotted. Uses include the following:

- *Patient monitoring and ventilator weaning in the ICU.* This is perhaps the most common use, particularly for patients who have been connected to the ventilator for days and in whom an arterial line is no longer being used. $PetCO_2$ is used as a proxy for $PaCO_2$ and, along with pulse oximetry, allows for safe ventilator monitoring and weaning. One aspect of such monitoring is heralding a ventilator disconnect. An alarm on the $PetCO_2$ monitor can tell if there is a disconnection, since the $PetCO_2$ will abruptly go to zero.

- *Patient monitoring during general anesthesia.* The principle is the same as when monitoring the ventilator in the ICU.
- *Indication of a sudden increase in dead space and, therefore, altered ventilation–perfusion in the lungs.* Virtually any condition that increases dead space can abruptly lower $PetCO_2$ (and thereby increase the difference between $PaCO_2$ and $PetCO_2$). One cause is reduction in blood perfusion to the lungs. Thus a sudden fall in cardiac output will be heralded by a fall in the $PetCO_2$, as less CO_2 is delivered to the lungs for excretion (Isserles 1991; Shibutani 1992; Shibutani 1994). Similarly, a rise in cardiac output will be accompanied by a rise in $PetCO_2$ (Fig. 3.7.).

Another perfusion-related cause of fall in $PetCO_2$ is acute pulmonary embolism (Eriksson et al. 1989; Hatle & Rokseth 1974). An embolus in the pulmonary circulation creates extra dead space by blocking perfusion to a group

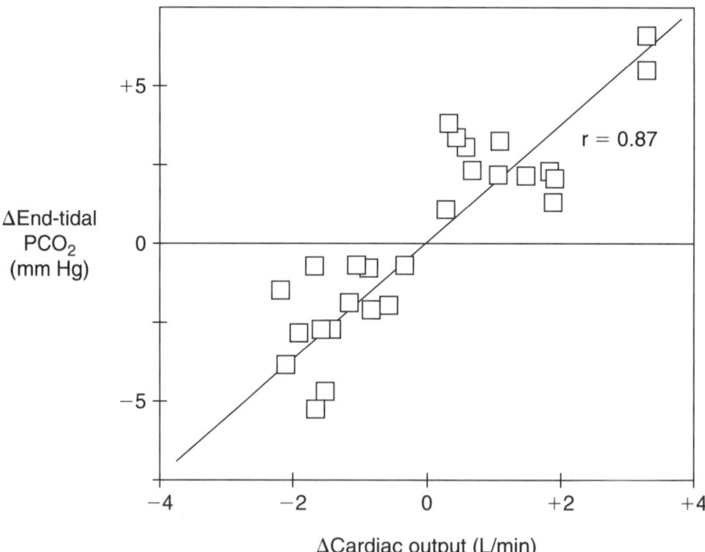

Figure 3.7. Correlation of changes in $PetCO_2$ with changes in cardiac output. Reprinted with permission from Shibutani 1992.

of alveoli (the same principle as illustrated in Fig. 3.5*B*). Air reaches these alveoli but does not take part in gas exchange (hence the creation of dead space) because perfusion is blocked. The acute increase in dead space is nonspecific, so a fall in $PetCO_2$ does not obviate obtaining more specific diagnostic studies.

- *Prediction of nonsurvival from cardiac arrest.* Several studies have shown that a persistently low $PetCO_2$ during CPR correlates with nonsurvival from cardiac arrest (Callaham & Barton 1990; Sanders et al. 1989; Wayne 1995). In a large study of victims of pulseless electrical activity, a $PetCO_2 < 10$ mm Hg after 20 min of CPR predicted nonsurvival; everyone who survived to hospital admission had a $PetCO_2 > 18$ mm Hg after 20 min of CPR (Levine et al. 1997; Fig. 3.8).

Clinical Problem 3.11. For each of the following conditions, state if the $PaCO_2$–$PetCO_2$ difference should be normal/near normal (N) or abnormal (A).

a. A 64-year-old man with severe emphysema
b. A 35-year-old woman with normal lungs who is hyperventilating, $PaCO_2 = 25$ mm Hg
c. A 24-year-old man with normal lungs who is hypoventilating from drug overdose, $PaCO_2 = 55$ mm Hg
d. A 42-year-old woman with a pulmonary embolism
e. A 78-year-old man with cardiogenic shock
f. A 30-year-old man with normal lungs, exercising on a treadmill at 5 mph for 10 min

THE RELATIONSHIP OF $PaCO_2$ TO OXYGENATION AND ACID–BASE BALANCE

Any discussion of gas exchange and arterial blood gases should begin with $PaCO_2$. $PaCO_2$ is the only blood gas value that provides information on ventilation, oxygenation, and acid–base balance. Figure 3.9 shows the relationship of $PaCO_2$ to

- Alveolar ventilation in the $PaCO_2$ equation (as discussed in this chapter)
- PAO_2 in the alveolar gas equation (see Chapter 4)
- pH in the Henderson–Hasselbalch equation (see Chapter 7).

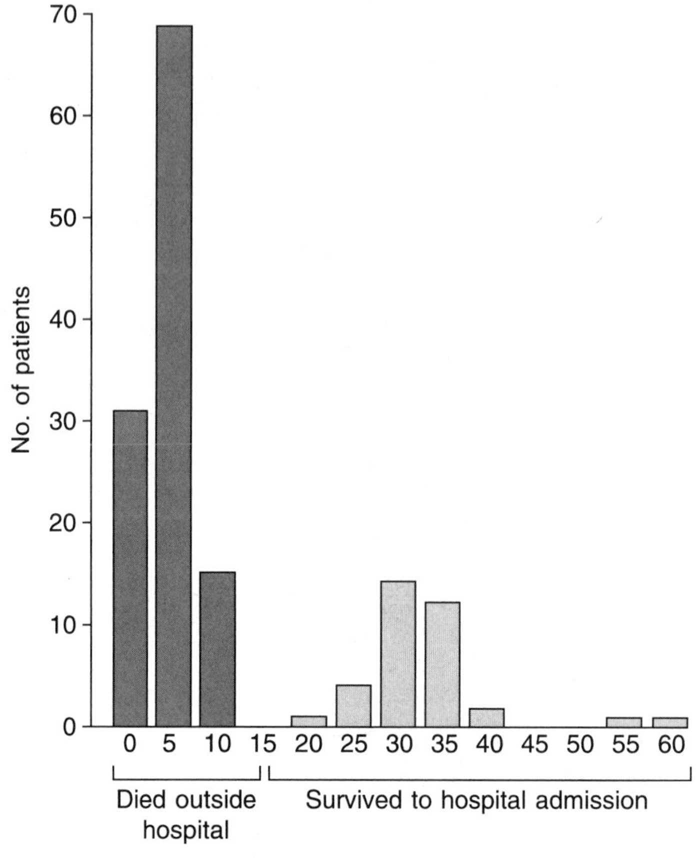

Figure 3.8. A low $PetCO_2$ predicts nonsurvival of out-of-hospital cardiac arrest. The number of patients is shown for each midpoint grouping of $PetCO_2$. All patients with a $PetCO_2 < 10$ mm Hg died outside of the hospital; all those with a $PetCO_2 > 18$ mm Hg survived to hospital admission. Reprinted with permission from Levine RL, Wayne MA, Miller CC. End-tidal carbon dioxide and outcome of out-of-hospital cardiac arrest. N Engl J Med 1997;337:301–306.

$PaCO_2$ is the key to understanding arterial blood gases in clinical practice. If you understand $PaCO_2$ and all its ramifications—the difference between alveolar and minute ventilation, what determines hyperventilation and hypoventilation, the role of $PaCO_2$ in the alveolar gas and H–H equations, and the utility of $PetCO_2$—you will be well on your way to mastering arterial blood gas interpretation.

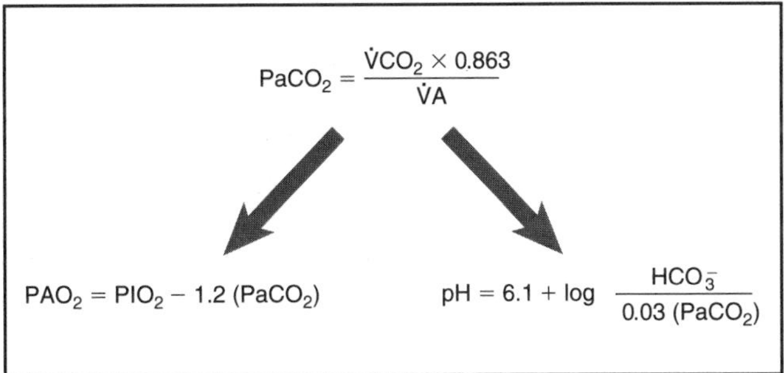

Figure 3.9. $PaCO_2$ in ventilation, oxygenation, and acid–base equations. An elevated $PaCO_2$ indicates diminished $\dot{V}A$ relative to $\dot{V}CO_2$ and will result in a fall in PAO_2 (and hence PaO_2) and pH.

ANSWERS TO CLINICAL PROBLEMS

3.1. The $\dot{V}E$ or minute ventilation is $12 \times 500 = 6$ L/min. We are told that $\dot{V}A = 3$ L/min. Hence $\dot{V}D = \dot{V}E - \dot{V}A = 3$ L/min. The dead space volume is one-twelfth of the dead space ventilation, or 250 mL.

3.2. Alveolar ventilation is that part of total ventilation that reaches the alveoli and takes part in gas exchange. By definition, what's left includes all the air that enters the airways and does not take part in gas exchange, a volume that makes up the physiologic dead space.

3.3. First, you must calculate the alveolar ventilation. Because minute ventilation is 24×300 or 7.2 L/min and dead space ventilation is 24×150 or 3.6 L/min, alveolar ventilation is 3.6 L/min. Then

$$PaCO_2 = \frac{\dot{V}CO_2 \times 0.863}{\dot{V}A}$$

$$PaCO_2 = \frac{300\ \text{mL/min} \times 0.863}{3.6\ \text{L/min}}$$

$$PaCO_2 = 71.9\ \text{mm Hg}$$

3.4. This patient is definitely hypoventilating.

3.5.

$$\dot{V}A = \dot{V}E - \dot{V}D$$
$$= 10(600) - 10(150)$$
$$= 6 - 1.5 = 4.5 \text{ L/min}$$

$$PaCO_2 = \frac{200 \text{ mL/min} \times 0.863}{4.5 \text{ L/min}} = 38.4 \text{ mm Hg}$$

3.6. This patient has normal alveolar ventilation for the rate of CO_2 production. However, the appearance of respiratory distress suggests the patient is trying to hyperventilate but can't, a potentially dangerous situation.

3.7. Of the examples presented, you have only enough information to state that patient b is hyperventilating. The other two patients may be hyperventilating but they might also be hypoventilating. Respiratory rate, tidal volume, and use of accessory muscles are not sufficient information to make this determination.

3.8. You could obtain the requested information from the graph shown in Figure 3.2 or calculate $PaCO_2$ using the $PaCO_2$ equation in each situation. The answers below are from actual calculations.

a. 30 mm Hg, $\dot{V}A$ = 8.63 L/min. A decrease in $\dot{V}A$ to 7.63 L/min will give a $PaCO_2$ of 33.0 mm Hg (increase of 3 mm Hg)
b. 40 mm Hg, $\dot{V}A$ = 6.47 L/min. A decrease of $\dot{V}A$ to 5.47 L/min will give a $PaCO_2$ of 47.3 mm Hg (increase of 7.3 mm Hg)
c. 50 mm Hg, $\dot{V}A$ = 5.18 L/min. A decrease of $\dot{V}A$ to 4.18 L/min will give a $PaCO_2$ of 61.9 mm Hg (an increase of 11.9 mm Hg)

3.9. In this problem, alveolar ventilation is fixed at 4 L/min; the $PaCO_2$ for different rates of CO_2 production are calculated using the $PaCO_2$ equation.

a. 200 mL/min; $PaCO_2$ = 43.2 mm Hg
b. 300 mL/min; $PaCO_2$ = 64.7 mm Hg
c. 400 mL/min; $PaCO_2$ = 86.3 mm Hg

3.10. Exercise increases CO_2 production. People with a normal respiratory system are always able to augment alveolar ventilation to meet or exceed the amount of $\dot{V}A$ necessary to excrete any excess CO_2 production. As in this example, patients with severe COPD or other forms of chronic lung disease are often not able to increase their alveolar ventilation. This patient's resting alveolar ventilation is

$$\frac{20 \text{ mL/min} \times 0.863}{40 \text{ mm Hg}} = 4.32 \text{ L/min}$$

Since he increased CO_2 production by 50% and alveolar ventilation not at all, his new $PaCO_2$ is

$$\frac{300 \text{ mL/min} \times 0.863}{4.32 \text{ L/min}} = 59.9 \text{ mm Hg}$$

3.11. Generally, people without ventilation–perfusion imbalance should have a normal $PaCO_2$–$PetCO_2$ difference. Thus

a. A
b. N
c. N
d. A
e. A
f. N

CHAPTER

4

PaO_2 and the Alveolar–Arterial PO_2 Difference

MEAN ALVEOLAR PO_2 AND THE ALVEOLAR GAS EQUATION

The principal function of the lungs is to exchange oxygen and carbon dioxide with the atmosphere. The lungs take in fresh air, a mixture of 21% oxygen, 78% nitrogen, and trace carbon dioxide, and exhale stale air, a mixture of 17% oxygen, 78% nitrogen, and about 4% carbon dioxide (Fig. 4.1).

Only CO_2 and O_2 participate in gas exchange; there is no net exchange for nitrogen or other inert gases. Exchange of CO_2 and O_2 takes place through the alveolar–capillary membrane by passive diffusion, from a region of relatively higher gas pressure to one of relatively lower gas pressure (Fig. 4.2). (In the early 20th century, there was debate about whether gas exchange involved active transport; experiments at various altitudes showed passive diffusion is the only physiologic process involved.)

The process of gas exchange illustrated in Figures 4.1 and 4.2 can be examined at any time by several readily available measurements (PaO_2, SaO_2, and hemoglobin content) and calculations (A–a PO_2 difference and arterial oxygen content). Understanding these measurements and calculations, and their relationships, is the subject of this and the next two chapters.

Since O_2 enters the pulmonary capillary blood by diffusion, alveolar PO_2 must be a major determinant of pulmonary capillary and arterial PO_2. By the same reasoning, PAO_2 defines the upper limit of PaO_2; PaO_2 can never be higher than PAO_2 if oxygen is to enter the blood. In the so-called ideal lung, PaO_2 would equal PAO_2. Gas exchange is not ideal, however, and so PaO_2 should *always be less* than the calculated PAO_2. The actual difference between calculated PAO_2 and measured PaO_2 depends on several factors, the most important of which is the relationship of ventilation to perfusion among the hundreds of millions alveolar–capillary units.

There are several hundred million individual alveoli. The PO_2 within their air spaces is not uniform, mainly because of effects of gravity and compliance. (In upright humans, compliance or distensibility of the lungs is lowest at the apices

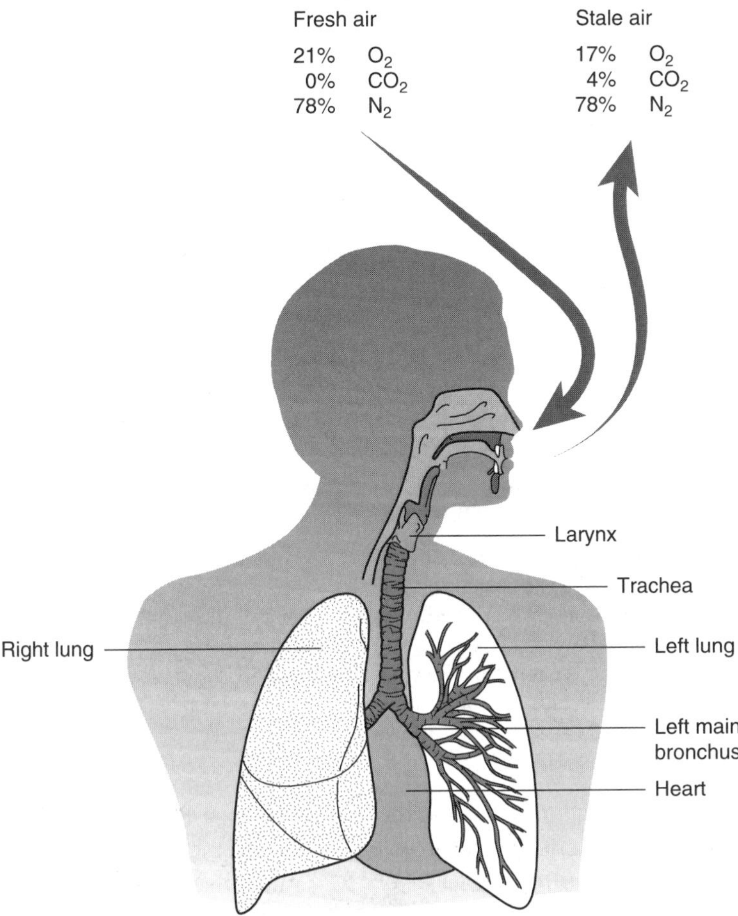

Figure 4.1. Gas exchange within the lungs. The differences between inhaled and exhaled O_2 and CO_2 represent gas exchange with the atmosphere.

and highest at the bases.) For clinical purposes we don't have to concern ourselves with the distribution of individual alveolar PO_2 values. We need to know only the average PO_2 of *all* the alveoli, a value obtained by the alveolar gas equation:

$$PAO_2 = PIO_2 - 1.2(PaCO_2)$$

where

$$PIO_2 = FIO_2(P_B - 47)$$

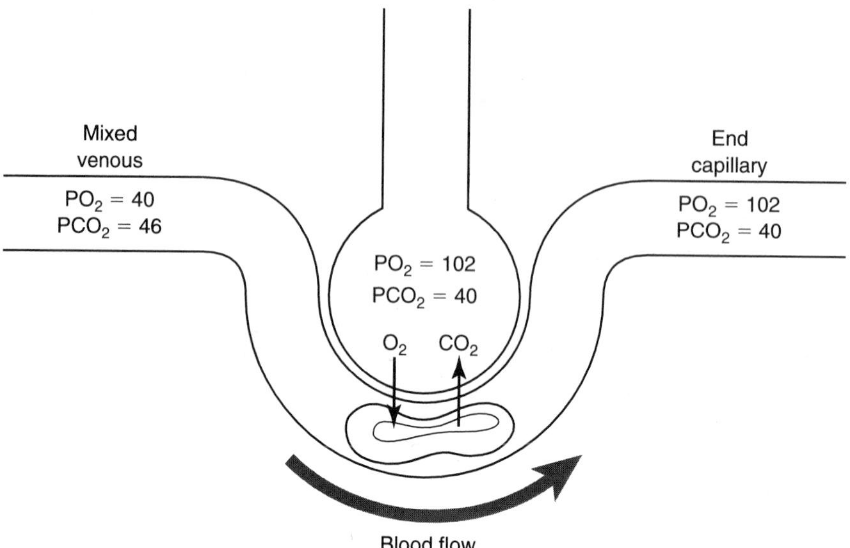

Figure 4.2. O_2 and CO_2 are exchanged through the alveolar–capillary membrane by diffusion from a region of relatively higher gas pressure to one of relatively lower gas pressure. Here, the difference between PCO_2 in blood entering the pulmonary capillary (mixed venous) and in the alveolus is 6 mm Hg. The difference between PO_2 in blood entering the pulmonary capillary and alveolus is 62 mm Hg. Note that end-capillary PO_2 and PCO_2 are identical to the alveolar PO_2 and PCO_2, respectively.

The alveolar gas equation states that the average alveolar PO_2 equals the inspired PO_2 minus the arterial PCO_2 (times 1.2). Although the alveolar gas equation is formally derived using *alveolar* PCO_2, we assume that $PaCO_2 = PACO_2$ (as with the PCO_2 equation).

The factor 1.2 accounts for the slight variation in nitrogen pressure as more O_2 is taken up than CO_2 is exhaled; the ratio of O_2 uptake to CO_2 exhaled is called the respiratory quotient and (for clinical purposes) is assumed to be 0.8. It is not necessary to measure RQ in the clinical setting (Cinel et al. 1991).

With increasing FIO_2, the multiplication factor decreases because nitrogen is being eliminated from the body. If there were complete denitrogenation of the alveoli and blood (by breathing 100% oxygen), the multiplication factor would become 1.0. In clinical practice, you can use the factor 1.2 up to an FIO_2 of 0.6 and then use 1.0 at 0.6 or higher inspired oxygen concentrations (Martin 1986).

In the calculation of PIO_2, water vapor pressure (47 mm Hg) is subtracted from barometric pressure to give dry gas pressure. Water vapor pressure varies slightly with body temperature, but the change is rarely enough to matter when calculating a patient's PAO_2.

Figure 4.3 shows measurements and calculations for PO_2 from the atmosphere to the mixed venous blood. The PaO_2 is determined by the alveolar PO_2 and the architecture of the lungs, which determines the amount of venous admixture. In Figure 4.3 the normal venous admixture of about 3% is illustrated by a shunt between the pulmonary arterial and pulmonary venous circulations (from some ventilation–perfusion imbalance within the lungs).

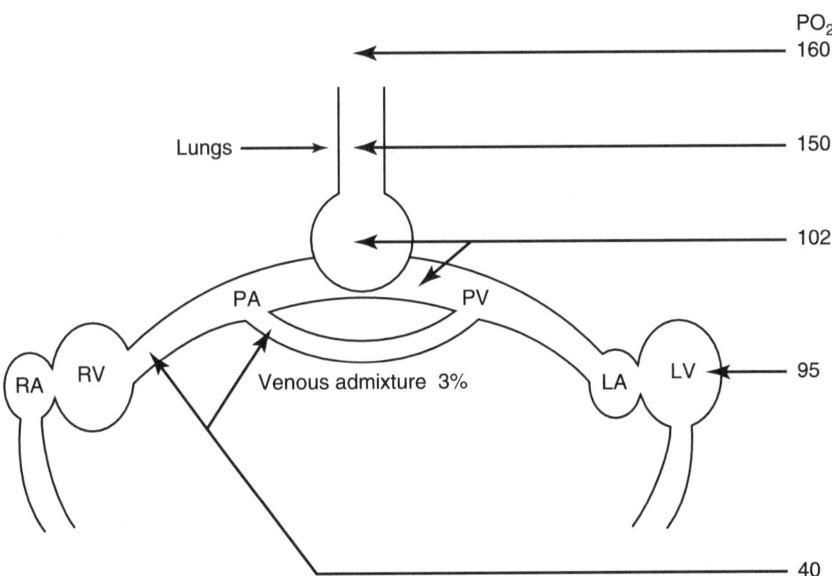

Figure 4.3. PO_2 from atmosphere to blood. The PaO_2 is determined by the alveolar PO_2 and the architecture of the lungs, defined as all factors that influence the air–capillary interface. The normal amount of ventilation–perfusion imbalance leads to a venous admixture of approximately 3%, i.e., 3% of the cardiac output is not oxygenated (illustrated by a shunt between the pulmonary arterial and pulmonary venous circulations). The PO_2 values assume a barometric pressure of 760 mm Hg, an FIO_2 of 0.21, and normal lungs. PO_2 values shown are: atmospheric, 160; tracheal, 150; alveolar, 102; arterial, 94; and venous, 40 mm Hg. PaO_2 is one of two major determinants of SaO_2; the other is the position of the oxygen dissociation curve (Chapter 6). Modified from Martin L. Pulmonary physiology in clinical practice. St. Louis: Mosby-Year Book, 1987. *RA,* right atrium; *PV,* pulmonary veins; *RV,* right ventricle; *LA,* left atrium; *PA,* pulmonary arteries; *LV,* left ventricle.

Clinical Problem 4.1. Which of the following will not lower the alveolar PO_2?

a. Increase in altitude
b. Elevated $PACO_2$
c. Increase in venous admixture
d. Breath holding

Clinical Problem 4.2. Which of the following will not raise the alveolar PO_2?

a. Increase in FIO_2
b. Increase in barometric pressure
c. Hyperventilation
d. Decrease in venous admixture

Ambient FIO_2 is 0.21 (or 21%) at all altitudes. For patients breathing supplemental oxygen, the correct FIO_2 must be known to obtain an accurate PAO_2. However, it is usually not necessary to measure barometric pressure (P_B) if you know its approximate average value where the blood was drawn (e.g., sea level = 760, Cleveland = 747, Denver = 640 mm Hg). This assumption facilitates calculation of PAO_2 because, for a given location, you can always use the same value for dry gas pressure. Table 4.1 shows gas pressures at several altitudes.

Note that PIO_2 in Table 4.1 refers to air in the trachea. At this point in the airway, water vapor has been added so that water vapor pressure (47 mm Hg) must be subtracted from the barometric pressure to obtain the PIO_2. In Chapter 1 we calculated the PO_2 in dry air and arrived at a figure of 134 mm Hg for Denver; once in the trachea, the PO_2 is 125 mm Hg.

What is the PIO_2 (in the trachea) of a patient breathing ambient air in Cleveland?

a. 147 mm Hg
b. 713 mm Hg
c. Must measure barometric pressure

While purists might answer c, the slight day-to-day variation in average barometric pressure is not critical to this calculation. In Cleveland, where the average P_B is about 747 mm Hg, the PIO_2 for a person breathing ambient (room) air is

$$0.21(747 - 47) = 147 \text{ mm Hg}$$

Do all these assumptions (about P_B, R value, water vapor pressure, etc.) weaken the validity of the alveolar gas equation? Not at all. Assumptions in clinical use for the alveolar gas equation (Table 4.2) allow PAO_2 to be readily calculated and used for patient assessment. It is always amusing to see someone report an alveolar–arterial PO_2 difference to the decimal point, e.g., 25.7 mm Hg; such precision is not only impossible to obtain, and therefore specious, it is clinically unnecessary.

TABLE 4.1. GAS PRESSURES AT VARIOUS ALTITUDES[a]

LOCATION	ALT	P_B	FIO_2	PIO_2	$PaCO_2$[b]	PAO_2	PAO_2[c]
Sea level	0	760	0.21	150	40	102	95
Cleveland	500	747	0.21	147	40	99	92
Denver	5,280	640	0.21	125	34	84	77
Pike's Peak	14,114	450	0.21	85	30	62	55
Mt. Everest	29,028	253	0.21	43	7.5	35	28

[a]All pressures in mm Hg.
[b]PAO_2 is calculated using an assumed R value of 0.8, except for the summit of Mt. Everest, for which 0.85 is used (West et al. 1983).
[c]Each PaO_2 value is normal for its respective altitude.
ALT, altitude in feet; *P_B*, barometric pressure; *FIO_2*, fraction of inspired oxygen; *PIO_2*, pressure of inspired oxygen in the trachea; *$PaCO_2$*, arterial PCO_2, assumed to be equal to alveolar PCO_2; *PAO_2*, alveolar PO_2; *PaO_2*, arterial PO_2, assuming a $P(A–a)O_2$ of 7 mm Hg at each altitude.

TABLE 4.2. ASSUMPTIONS VS. CLINICAL REALITY IN USE OF THE ALVEOLAR GAS EQUATION

ASSUMPTION	CLINICAL REALITY
Accurate P_B is known at the time blood is drawn	P_B is usually measured only once a day and may fluctuate throughout the day
RQ is 0.8	RQ is almost never measured, yet it can vary
$PaCO_2 = PACO_2$	In lung disease, $PaCO_2$ is often $\neq PACO_2$
Water vapor pressure is 47 mm Hg	Vapor pressure changes with body temperature
Accurate FIO_2 is known when the patient is breathing supplemental oxygen	FIO_2 is usually not precise unless the patient is using a specific type of face mask (Venturi) or is connected to a mechanical ventilator

Clinical Problem 4.3. What is the tracheal PIO_2 at sea level when the FIO_2 is 0.40?

a. 100 mm Hg
b. 150 mm Hg
c. 200 mm Hg
d. 285 mm Hg
e. Indeterminate without additional information

Clinical Problem 4.4. What is the PAO_2 at sea level in the following circumstances?

a. $FIO_2 = 1.00$; $PaCO_2 = 30$ mm Hg
b. $FIO_2 = 0.21$; $PaCO_2 = 50$ mm Hg
c. $FIO_2 = 0.40$; $PaCO_2 = 30$ mm Hg

Clinical Problem 4.5. What is the PAO_2 on the summit of Mount Everest in the following circumstances?

a. $FIO_2 = 0.21$; $PaCO_2 = 40$ mm Hg
b. $FIO_2 = 1.00$; $PaCO_2 = 40$ mm Hg
c. $FIO_2 = 0.21$; $PaCO_2 = 10$ mm Hg

THE ALVEOLAR–ARTERIAL PO_2 DIFFERENCE

By comparing the *calculated* PAO_2 with the *measured* PaO_2, we can learn much useful information about the patient's state of gas exchange. As already pointed out, PaO_2 should always be lower than PAO_2. The *difference* between the two PO_2 values depends on several factors, particularly the distribution of ventilation to perfusion among the millions of alveolar–capillary units.

It is important to distinguish between *diffusion block* and *ventilation–perfusion imbalance* as physiologic causes of hypoxemia. Both processes affect oxygen transfer from air into blood, but only the latter process plays a clinically significant role in hypoxemia.

Diffusion is the physiologic mechanism by which gas moves across a membrane, from a region of higher to one of lower pressure; it describes the movement of oxygen from the individual alveolar spaces across the alveolar–capillary membrane and into the pulmonary capillary blood, and the movement of CO_2 in the opposite direction.

Both oxygen and carbon dioxide diffuse across the alveolar–capillary membrane because of their respective pressure differences between alveolus and capillary blood. Diffusion of either gas is so rapid and efficient that any lung disease manifested by a "diffusion barrier" (e.g., pulmonary fibrosis, congestive heart failure) does not cause significant hypoxemia in patients at rest.

Diffusion block *may* cause hypoxemia under certain circumstances, e.g., exercise in patients with interstitial fibrosis. With CO_2, diffusion impairment is *never* a cause of CO_2 retention under any circumstances. It is a common misconception to attribute CO_2 retention to a diffusion block; patients retain CO_2 because of underventilation of alveoli, never because of diffusion impairment.

The term *ventilation–perfusion* (V–Q) refers to the amount of air entering the alveoli per minute *relative* to the capillary perfusion of those alveoli. A V–Q ratio of 1.0 means that an amount of ventilation in an alveolar unit (e.g., 1 mL/min) is available to exchange gases with an equal amount of capillary blood in that unit (1 mL/min). Equality of ventilation to perfusion is the ideal. Figure 4.4 shows the range of V–Q ratios.

V–Q imbalance occurs when there is more or less ventilation for the amount of perfusion. For example, if there is twice as much ventilation in an alveolus for the amount of capillary perfusion, the V–Q ratio of that unit is 2.0; if there is half as much ventilation as perfusion, the V–Q ratio is 0.5, etc.

In the normal upright lung, apical alveoli have high V–Q ratios and basilar alveoli have low V–Q ratios. High V–Q ratios result in alveolar dead space (physiologic dead space) and wasted ventilation (see Chapter 3); blood leaving these units has a relatively high PO_2 and low PCO_2. Low V–Q ratios result in underventilation and pulmonary capillary blood that is poorly oxygenated, or venous admixture (venous blood is admixed with normally oxygenated blood). Compared to the average for the lungs, blood leaving low V–Q units has a relatively low PO_2 and a relatively high PCO_2 (Fig. 4.4).

Note that blood perfusing alveolar units with no ventilation gives those units a V–Q ratio of zero. This is colloquially called a "shunt"; the correct terminology is *right-to-left shunt of pulmonary capillary blood.* V–Q units of zero have the same

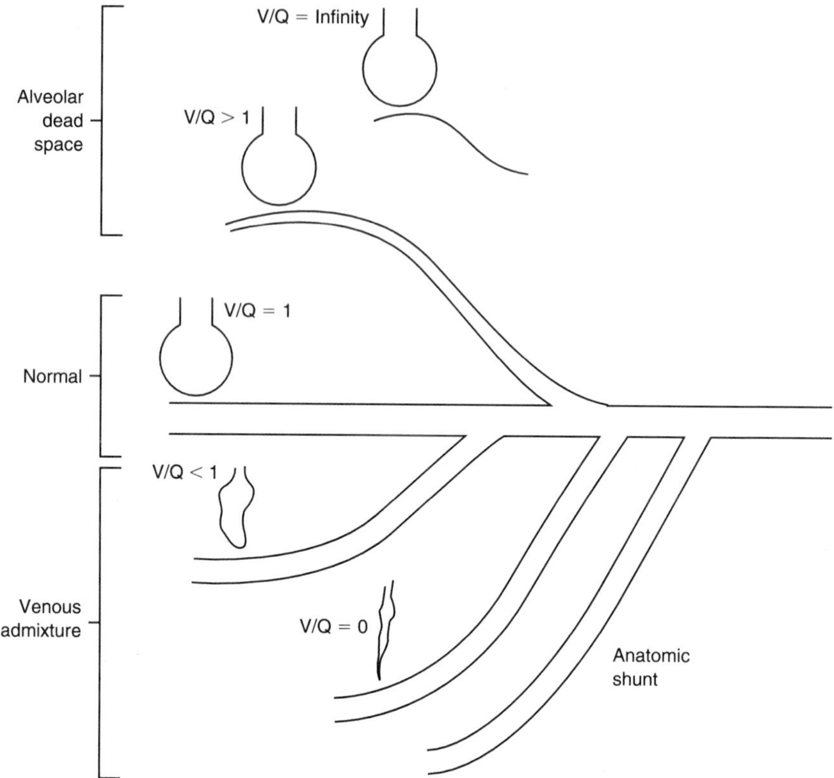

Figure 4.4. The range of V–Q ratios. Alveolar–capillary units with low V–Q ratios represent venous admixture. Units with high V–Q ratios represent alveolar dead space.

effect on oxygenation as if the blood were shunted anatomically (e.g., through an arterial-venous fistula). A shunt, therefore, is really an extreme of V–Q imbalance. No amount of inhaled O_2 can oxygenate shunted blood; whereas given a high enough FIO_2 and time, blood perfusing low V–Q units can become oxygenated.

Although normal lungs have both high and low V–Q units, the V–Q ratios tend to balance, so that the *overall* V–Q distribution of the normal lungs approaches 1.0. Even so, the overventilated units cannot compensate fully for underoxygenation resulting from the low or zero V–Q units. For this reason, the arterial PO_2 ends up slightly lower than the alveolar PO_2. This normal difference between alveolar and arterial PO_2 is the result of V–Q inequality and *not* to any diffusion barrier.

Given a normal V–Q ratio, the PO_2 of blood leaving the alveolus (end-capillary PO_2) is almost identical to the alveolar PO_2 (Fig. 4.2). An alveolar–arterial PO_2 difference arises because in the lungs some units are underventilated for the amount of blood perfusing them; when blood leaving these units mixes with the overoxygenated blood from high V–Q units, the result is invariably a PO_2 lower than the mean alveolar PO_2. Simply stated, the greater the degree of V–Q imbalance, the worse the hypoxemia. (As long as there is sufficient alveolar ventilation, CO_2 will be unaffected by degrees of V–Q imbalance that routinely lead to hypoxemia).

The term *A–a gradient* is really a misnomer, because the difference between mean alveolar PO_2 and arterial PO_2 is the result of V–Q imbalance or diffusion impairment, not to any oxygen gradient between alveolus and pulmonary capillary blood. The physiologically correct term is *A–a O_2 difference*. This difference—one of oxygen pressures—will be written here as $P(A–a)O_2$.

If there were no V–Q imbalance the $P(A–a)O_2$ would be

a. Same as with a V–Q imbalance
b. Almost zero

If there were no V–Q imbalance, the $P(A–a)O_2$ would be almost zero. The difference between alveolar and end-capillary PO_2 is negligible when ventilation matches perfusion and the alveolar–capillary membrane is of normal thickness; diffusion of oxygen across the membrane is "complete" in normal lungs. A finite $P(A–a)O_2$ exists because the V–Q imbalance in healthy lungs (a result mainly of gravity) leads to some low V–Q units, i.e., units with relatively poorer ventilation for the amount of perfusion; this situation occurs mainly in the lung bases.

These low V–Q units result in a reduced end-capillary PO_2; this, in turn, depresses the arterial PO_2 to a level below the mean alveolar PO_2 value. Without any V–Q imbalance (a nonexistent ideal) the average of *all* end-capillary PO_2 values—and hence the arterial PO_2—would equal the mean alveolar PO_2.

The normal range for $P(A–a)O_2$ is

a. 5–15 mm Hg for young to middle-aged people breathing room air (FIO_2 = 0.21)
b. 15–25 mm Hg for elderly people (FIO_2 = 0.21)

c. 10–110 mm Hg for individuals breathing 100% oxygen
d. All of the above

Although normal $P(A-a)O_2$ is sometimes quoted as 5–15 mm Hg, that is true only for the conditions specified in answer a. Elderly people have a higher normal $P(A-a)O_2$ (Fig. 4.5). Sorbini et al. (1968) calculated the relationship (for healthy supine individuals) as $PaO_2 = 109 - 0.43$(age in years). Finally, since $P(A-a)O_2$ varies with FIO_2 (Fig. 4.6), all choices are correct.

ARE THE LUNGS TRANSFERRING OXYGEN PROPERLY? THE CLINICAL USEFULNESS OF $P(A-a)O_2$

If PIO_2 is held constant and $PaCO_2$ increases, PAO_2 (and PaO_2) will always decrease. Since PAO_2 is calculated based on known (or assumed) factors, its change is predictable. PaO_2, by contrast, is a measurement with a theoretical maximum value defined by PAO_2, and the actual value is determined by the state of the

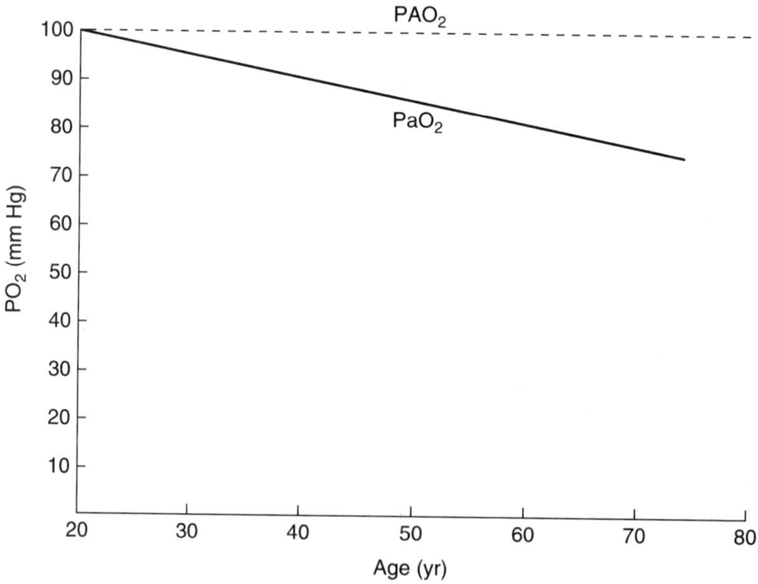

Figure 4.5. Decline of PaO_2 and increase in $P(A-a)O_2$ with increasing age. PaO_2 data from Sorbini CA, Grassi B, Solinas E, Muiesan G. Arterial oxygen tension in relation to age in healthy subjects. Respiration 1968;25:3–13.

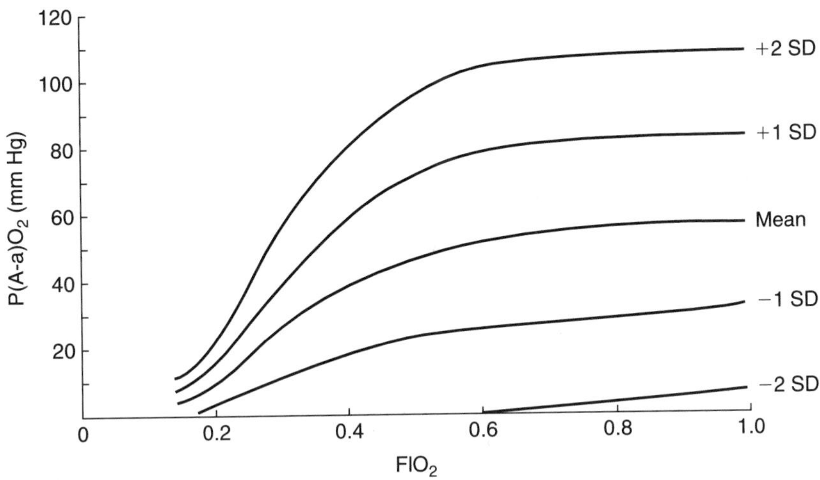

Figure 4.6. Normal range of $P(A–a)O_2$ from FIO_2 of 0.21 to 1.00, based on data obtained from 16 healthy subjects aged 40–50 years. Lines represent mean values ±2 standard deviations (*SD*). $P(A–a)O_2$ increases with increasing FIO_2 up to 0.6 and then reaches a plateau with further increases in FIO_2. Note that the $P(A–a)O_2$ may normally exceed 100 mm Hg when FIO_2 is 1.00. Reprinted with permission from Harris EA, Kenyon AM, Nisbet HD, et al. The normal alveolar–arterial oxygen tension gradient in man. Clin Sci Mol Med 1974;46:89–104.

CASE. *A 27-year-old woman comes to the emergency department complaining of pleuritic chest pain. She has been taking birth control pills. Her chest x-ray and physical exam are normal. Arterial blood gas shows pH = 7.45, $PaCO_2$ = 31 mm Hg, HCO_3^- = 21 mEq/L, PaO_2 = 83 mm Hg (FIO_2 = 0.21; P_B = 747 mm Hg). Viral pleurodynia is presumptively diagnosed, and she is discharged home with a prescription for pain medication.*

ventilation–perfusion imbalance, cardiac output, and O_2 content of blood entering the pulmonary artery (mixed venous blood). In particular, the greater the imbalance of ventilation–perfusion ratios, the more PaO_2 tends to differ from the calculated PAO_2.

What was this patient's PIO_2, PAO_2, $P(A–a)O_2$, and PaO_2/FIO_2 in the emergency room?

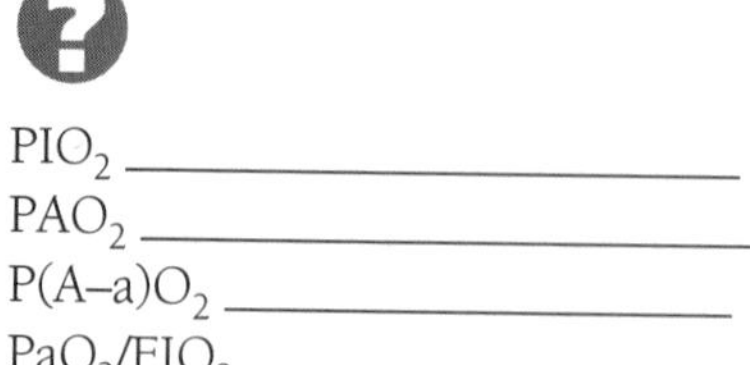

PIO_2 ____________________
PAO_2 ____________________
$P(A–a)O_2$ ____________________
PaO_2/FIO_2 ____________________

This young woman's PaO_2 was initially judged normal, and her defect in oxygen transfer went unappreciated. The calculated PIO_2 and PAO_2 were 147 and 110 mm Hg, respectively; thus her $P(A–a)O_2$ was elevated at 27 mm Hg (110 – 83), indicating gas transfer abnormality. She returned the next day with similar complaints; a lung scan was done and interpreted as "high probability" for pulmonary embolism (PE). PE was no doubt the cause of her increased $P(A–a)O_2$ when she was first seen.

As this case illustrates, the principal value of calculating PAO_2 is to allow for proper interpretation of a given PaO_2. Let's say you have a blood gas result showing a PaO_2 of 55 mm Hg. Why is it lower than normal? From low barometric pressure? Low FIO_2? Hypoventilation? Or does the low PaO_2 represent a gas exchange defect within the lungs (and, therefore, a ventilation–perfusion imbalance)? Answers to these everyday clinical questions can often be obtained by calculating the alveolar PO_2 and the alveolar–arterial PO_2 difference.

One cannot properly assess *any* PaO_2 without knowing, at minimum, the barometric pressure, FIO_2, and $PaCO_2$, information incorporated in the equation for PAO_2. Consider the following three PaO_2 values: 95, 60, and 28. Based solely on the normal range for PaO_2, the first value seems normal and the other two reduced, the last one critically so; however, do any of the three values represent a problem with gas exchange? From these values alone could you decide if the lungs are working properly? Could the "normal" PaO_2 reflect a serious gas exchange problem? Could there be *no* gas exchange problem with the other two values?

Under what circumstance could a PaO_2 of 95 mm Hg represent severe gas exchange abnormality?

A PaO_2 of 95 mm Hg would be abnormal in anyone breathing 100% oxygen (unless the barometric pressure was very low).

What should the PaO_2 be in a 42-year-old man inhaling pure oxygen? Assume normal $P(A–a)O_2$ of 100 mm Hg on this FIO_2, normal ventilation, and a barometric pressure of 760 mm Hg.

a. 100 mm Hg
b. 250 mm Hg
c. > 550 mm Hg

Using the alveolar gas equation we find that

$$PAO_2 = 1.00\ (760 - 47) - 40 \text{ mm Hg} = 673 \text{ mm Hg}$$

If his PaO_2 was only 95 mm Hg, $P(A–a)O_2$ would be 578 mm Hg and would signify a marked gas exchange problem and a critical illness, e.g., pulmonary edema or acute respiratory distress syndrome. Without the additional information provided by the PAO_2 calculation, there is no way to assess whether a PaO_2 of 95 mm Hg reflects normal or abnormal gas exchange.

Under what circumstances could a PaO_2 of 60 mm Hg represent no gas exchange abnormality?

Again, you need to know the FIO_2, barometric pressure, and $PaCO_2$; any one of these three factors could reduce PAO_2 without any defect in the gas exchange function of the lungs.

What is the $P(A–a)O_2$ of a 35-year-old woman who took an overdose of sleeping pills and has a $PaCO_2$ of 65 mm Hg and a PaO_2 of 60 mm Hg? Assume barometric pressure is 760 mm Hg and the patient is breathing ambient air.

Using the alveolar gas equation we find that

$$PAO_2 = 0.21\ (713) - 1.2(65) = 72 \text{ mm Hg}$$

Since PaO_2 is 60 mm Hg, the $P(A–a)O_2$ is 12 mm Hg, a normal value. The patient is globally hypoventilating because of the drug overdose, but she has no problem with exchanging oxygen within her lungs. The normal $P(A–a)O_2$ suggests normal lung function in terms of gas exchange and that the problem (at this point) is hypoventilation from central nervous system depression.

If, under identical circumstances, her PaO_2 was measured at 40 mm Hg, then $P(A–a)O_2$ would be 32 mm Hg, and you would want to search for a pulmonary condition (such as aspiration pneumonia or pulmonary edema) to explain the defect in gas exchange.

Under what circumstances could a healthy individual have a PaO_2 of 28 mm Hg?

Again, you have to know the FIO_2, barometric pressure, and $PaCO_2$. A very low FIO_2 could explain this PaO_2. A subject breathing an FIO_2 of only 8% would have a PIO_2 of 57 mm Hg at sea level; with hyperventilation, for example to 20 mm Hg, the calculated alveolar PO_2 would be about 33 mm Hg and the $P(A–a)O_2$, 5 mm Hg. The problem in such a case is not with pulmonary gas exchange but the environment.

A PaO_2 of 28 mm Hg would also be normal under ambient conditions on the summit of Mount Everest, where barometric pressure is only 253 mm Hg and PIO_2 only 43 mm Hg (Table 4.1). To survive without supplemental oxygen at the summit (a feat accomplished by several people), the climber must hyperventilate markedly. If the climber maintained $PaCO_2$ at 40 mm Hg, his PAO_2 would be *minus* 5 mm Hg, a value wholly incompatible with life!

On one expedition to the summit, 10 min after supplemental O_2 was removed, a climber's end-tidal PCO_2 (equivalent to $PACO_2$) was measured at 7.5 mm Hg. The calculated PAO_2 was only 35 mm Hg. Based on a theoretical $P(A–a)O_2$ of 7 mm Hg, West et al. (1983) determined the climber's PaO_2 at the summit to be an astonishing 28 mm Hg—extremely low but "normal" for the circumstances.

In summary, to properly interpret PaO_2 one needs to know PAO_2, a calculation based on barometric pressure; FIO_2; water vapor pressure; and $PaCO_2$.

Clinical Problem 4.6. For each of the following scenarios, calculate the $P(A–a)O_2$ using the abbreviated alveolar gas equation; assume $P_B = 760$ mm Hg. Which of these patients is most likely to have lung disease? Do any of the values represent a measurement or recording error?

a. A 35-year-old man with $PaCO_2 = 50$ mm Hg and $PaO_2 = 150$ mm Hg; $FIO_2 = 0.40$
b. A 44-year-old woman with $PaCO_2 = 75$ mm Hg and $PaO_2 = 95$ mm Hg; $FIO_2 = 0.28$
c. A young, anxious man with $PaO_2 = 120$ mm Hg and $PaCO_2 = 15$ mm Hg; $FIO_2 = 0.21$
d. A woman in the intensive care unit with $PaO_2 = 350$ mm Hg and $PaCO_2 = 40$ mm Hg; $FIO_2 = 0.80$
e. A man with $PaO_2 = 80$ mm Hg and $PaCO_2 = 72$ mm Hg; FIO_2 0.21

PaO_2/FIO_2 AND OTHER INDICES OF HYPOXEMIA

Although the concept of $P(A–a)O_2$ is physiologically sound and is widely used, it presents two problems in actual clinical practice:

1. Normal $P(A–a)O_2$ varies significantly with FIO_2, ranging from about 5 to 15 mm Hg for room air up to > 100 mm Hg for 100% oxygen.
2. $P(A–a)O_2$ is rather cumbersome to calculate, even when one makes all the assumptions listed in Table 4.2.

Thus other indices of hypoxemia have been examined for clinical utility, including

- PaO_2/FIO_2
- PaO_2/PAO_2
- $P(A–a)O_2/PaO_2$

Of these three indices, only the PaO_2/FIO_2 is simpler than the $P(A–a)O_2$ (since the other two indices still require calculation of PAO_2). But does the PaO_2/FIO_2 also vary with FIO_2? The answer turns out to be, not as much as $P(A–a)O_2$. Although all the indices of hypoxemia listed above, including the $P(A–a)O_2$, vary with FIO_2, the PaO_2/FIO_2 exhibits the most stability at FIO_2 values ≥ 0.5 and PaO_2 values ≤ 100 mm Hg (Gowda & Klocke 1997).

For these reasons, simplicity and less variability with FIO_2 than the time-honored $P(A–a)O_2$, the PaO_2/FIO_2 has become the preferred index of hypoxemia to follow in critically ill patients.

The normal value for PaO_2/FIO_2 is

$$100/0.21 = 480$$

A ratio < 300 indicates a severe defect in gas exchange, and a value < 200 meets the criteria for acute respiratory distress syndrome (in the appropriate clinical setting, i.e., bilateral lung infiltrates of acute onset and not due to heart failure).

PaO_2/FIO_2 varies with FIO_2, but not as much as $P(A–a)O_2$. One problem with PaO_2/FIO_2 is that it doesn't account for changes in $PaCO_2$. The ratio can be misleading when the major reason for hypoxemia is hypercapnia or there is an increased $P(A–a)O_2$ with hyperventilation. However, if $PaCO_2$ is reasonably stable, PaO_2/FIO_2 is a useful parameter to follow in patients with varying PaO_2 and FIO_2.

What are the values for PaO_2/FIO_2 and $P(A–a)O_2$, in subjects breathing room air at sea level, when

a. $PaO_2 = 90$ mm Hg and $PaCO_2 = 20$ mm Hg
b. $PaO_2 = 66$ mm Hg and $PaCO_2 = 70$ mm Hg

In the first case, the PaO_2/FIO_2 is 429, which is normal; but the $P(A–a)O_2$ is abnormal at 36 mm Hg. In case b, the $P(A–a)O_2$ is normal at 7 mm Hg but the PaO_2/FIO_2 is abnormal at 280. Thus, for an isolated blood gas when $PaCO_2$ is abnormal, $P(A–a)O_2$ is apt to be more useful for determining if the lungs are transferring oxygen properly. The simplicity of the ratio, however, makes it more useful in following the progress of patients with severe hypoxemia whose $PaCO_2$ is not changing to any significant degree. Whatever index is used for this purpose, one should always be asking: Are the lungs transferring oxygen properly?

WHAT IS THE IMPLICATION OF AN ABNORMAL $P(A–a)O_2$ OR PaO_2/FIO_2?

If a 35-year-old man presents to the emergency department with a PaO_2 of 55 mm Hg at sea level and breathing room air, obviously he is hypoxemic. You don't need to calculate $P(A–a)O_2$ or PaO_2/FIO_2 to make this determination.

But in many situations, the PaO_2 will be above 80 mm Hg while the patient is breathing supplemental oxygen; then it is important to know if the $P(A–a)O_2$ is elevated or if PaO_2/FIO_2 is reduced. If so, the patient has a defect in gas exchange; some portion of the pulmonary circulation is inadequately oxygenated. The problem can be considered of *pulmonary* origin: i.e., an abnormal lung condition interfering with gas exchange. (A relatively uncommon nonpulmonary cause would be a right-to-left intracardiac shunt; this can usually be ruled out by clinical exam and echocardiography.)

Physiologic causes of a low PaO_2 are listed in Table 4.3. Although four respiratory and three nonrespiratory causes are listed, a low PaO_2 without elevated $PaCO_2$ is almost always the result of a V–Q imbalance and its variant, right-to-left shunting. A low mixed venous O_2 content can depress the PaO_2 if there is a concomitant severe V–Q imbalance or a right-to-left shunt.

TABLE 4.3. PHYSIOLOGIC CAUSES OF A LOW PaO_2.

	EFFECT ON	
PHYSIOLOGIC CAUSE[a]	$P(A–a)O_2$	PaO_2/FIO_2
Respiratory causes		
Pulmonary right-to-left shunt	Increased	Decreased
Severe pneumonia, ARDS, anatomic artery-to-vein shunt		
Ventilation–perfusion imbalance	Increased	Decreased
Parenchymal lung disease (asthma, pneumonia, pulmonary embolism, atelectasis)		
Diffusion barrier	Increased	Decreased
Interstitial fibrosis		
Hypoventilation (↑$PaCO_2$)	Normal	Decreased
Respiratory (ventilatory) failure		
Nonrespiratory causes		
Cardiac right-to-left shunt	Increased	Decreased
Ventricular septal defect, patent foramen ovale		
Decreased PIO_2	Normal	Normal
Decreased FIO_2, decreased barometric pressure		
Low mixed venous O_2 content[b]	Increased	Decreased
Severe anemia, cardiac failure		

[a]Clinical examples are listed below each cause.
[b]In the presence of an increased right-to-left shunt.
PIO_2, pressure of inspired oxygen; *FIO_2*, fraction of inspired oxygen; *ARDS*, acute respiratory distress syndrome.

ANSWERS TO CLINICAL PROBLEMS

4.1. c. Increase in venous admixture. The other choices will all lower the PAO_2. Breath holding reduces PAO_2 because oxygen is being taken up from the alveoli and not replenished.

4.2. d. Decrease in venous admixture. The other choices will all raise the PAO_2. Factors that influence alveolar PO_2 are inherent in the PAO_2 equation: barometric pressure (which varies with altitude), FIO_2, and $PACO_2$. Factors in the blood don't affect PAO_2, with one exception: $PaCO_2$. An increased $PaCO_2$ will increase $PACO_2$ and lower PAO_2. Hyperventilation reduces $PACO_2$ first; as a result, PAO_2 increases.

4.3. PIO_2 refers to the tracheal PO_2, so water vapor must be subtracted from the sea level barometric pressure of 760 mm Hg. The FIO_2 is given as 0.40. Hence

$$PIO_2 = 0.40(760 - 47) = 285 \text{ mm Hg}$$

4.4. To calculate PAO_2, the $PaCO_2$ must be subtracted from the PIO_2. Again, the barometric pressure is 760 mm Hg, since the values are obtained at sea level. In case a, the $PaCO_2$ of 30 mm Hg is not multiplied by 1.2, since the FIO_2 is 1.00. In cases b and c, the factor 1.2 is multiplied times the $PaCO_2$.

a. $PAO_2 = 1.00(713) - 30 = 683$ mm Hg
b. $PAO_2 = 0.21(713) - 1.2(50) = 90$ mm Hg
c. $PAO_2 = 0.40(713) - 1.2(30) = 249$ mm Hg

4.5. The PAO_2 on the summit of Mount Everest is calculated just as at sea level, using the barometric pressure of 253 mm Hg. (Although the respiratory quotient is not known—West et al. (1983) assumed a value of 0.85—you can use the same abbreviated equation as in problem 4.4.)

a. $PAO_2 = 0.21(253 - 47) - 1.2(40) = -5$ mm Hg
b. $PAO_2 = 1.00(253 - 47) - 40 = 166$ mm Hg
c. $PAO_2 = 0.21(253 - 47) - 1.2(10) = 31$ mm Hg

4.6. You are asked to calculate the $P(A\text{–}a)O_2$ for five different patients.

a.

$$PAO_2 = 0.40\,(760 - 47) - 1.2(50) = 225 \text{ mm Hg}$$
$$P(A\text{–}a)O_2 = 225 - 150 = 75 \text{ mm Hg}$$

The $P(A\text{–}a)O_2$ is elevated but still within the normal range for this FIO_2 (Fig. 4.6), so the patient may or may not have a defect in gas exchange.

b.

$PAO_2 = 0.28(713) - 1.2(75) = 200 - 90 = 110$ mm Hg
$P(A–a)O_2 = 110 - 95 = 15$ mm Hg

Despite severe hypoventilation, there is no evidence for *lung* disease. Hypercapnia is most likely a result of disease elsewhere in the respiratory system, either the central nervous system or the chest bellows.

c.

$PAO_2 = 0.21(713) - 1.2(15) = 150 - 18 = 132$ mm Hg
$P(A–a)O_2 = 132 - 120 = 12$ mm Hg

Hyperventilation can easily raise PaO_2 above 100 mm Hg when the lungs are normal, as in this case.

d.

$PAO_2 = 0.80\ (713) - 40 = 530$ mm Hg (Note that the factor 1.2 is dropped since $FIO_2 > 60\%$)
$P(A–a)O_2 = 530 - 350 = 180$ mm Hg

Despite a very high PaO_2, the lungs are not transferring oxygen normally.

e.

$PAO_2 = 0.21\ (713) - 1.2(72) = 150 - 86 = 64$ mm Hg
$P(A–a)O_2 = 64 - 80 = -16$ mm Hg

A negative $P(A–a)O_2$ is incompatible with life (unless there has been a sudden fall in FIO_2, which is not the case here). In this example, the negative $P(A–a)O_2$ can be explained by any of the following: incorrect FIO_2, incorrect blood gas measurement, or a reporting or transcription error.

CHAPTER

5 PaO_2, SaO_2, and Oxygen Content

HOW MUCH OXYGEN IS IN THE BLOOD?

In Chapter 4 you learned how to assess PaO_2 as an indicator of pulmonary gas exchange by comparing it with the alveolar PO_2 (PAO_2). You learned that a PaO_2 of 50 mm Hg could reflect no lung problem whatsoever under some circumstances, such as at high altitude where low barometric pressure causes reduction of both PAO_2 and PaO_2. And, similarly, a PaO_2 of 90 mm Hg could reflect severe gas exchange defect if the FIO_2 and PAO_2 are very high.

In addition to assessing adequacy of gas exchange within the lungs, it is important to assess adequacy of the blood's oxygen levels; simply put, is there sufficient oxygen for the patient? The PaO_2, or *oxygen pressure,* is, of course, one of the values used to characterize blood oxygen levels; however, two other values are more useful for this purpose: *oxygen saturation* and *oxygen content.* These three terms will be briefly defined, and then I will present a more detailed discussion of each, emphasizing their interrelationships.

Oxygen pressure: PaO_2. Oxygen molecules dissolved in plasma (i.e., not bound to hemoglobin) are free to impinge on the measuring oxygen electrode. This impingement of free O_2 molecules is reflected as the partial pressure of oxygen; if the sample being tested is arterial blood, then it is the PaO_2. Although the number of O_2 molecules dissolved in plasma determines, along with other factors, how many molecules will bind to hemoglobin, *once bound the oxygen molecules no longer exert any pressure* (bound oxygen molecules are no longer free to impinge on the measuring electrode). Because PaO_2 reflects only free oxygen molecules dissolved in plasma and not those bound to hemoglobin, PaO_2 cannot tell us how much oxygen is in the blood; for that you need to know how much oxygen is also bound to hemoglobin, information given by the SaO_2 and hemoglobin content.

Oxygen saturation: SaO_2. Binding sites for oxygen are the heme groups, the Fe^{++}-porphyrin portions of the hemoglobin molecule. There are four heme sites, and hence four oxygen-binding sites, per hemoglobin molecule. Heme sites occupied by oxygen molecules are said to be saturated with oxygen. The percentage of all the available heme-binding sites saturated with oxygen is the hemoglobin oxygen saturation (in arterial blood, the SaO_2). Note that SaO_2 alone doesn't reveal how much oxygen is in the blood; for that we also need to know the hemoglobin content.

Oxygen content: CaO_2. Tissues need a requisite amount of O_2 molecules for metabolism. Neither the PaO_2 nor the SaO_2 provide information on the number of oxygen molecules (i.e., how much oxygen) is in the blood. (Note that neither the PaO_2 nor the SaO_2 have units that denote any quantity.) Of the three values used for assessing blood oxygen levels, "how much" is provided only by the oxygen content, CaO_2 (unit = mL O_2/dL). This is because CaO_2 is the only value that incorporates the hemoglobin content. Oxygen content can be measured directly or calculated by the oxygen content equation (introduced in Chapter 2):

$$CaO_2 = \text{Hb (g/dL)} \times 1.34 \text{ mL } O_2\text{/g Hb} \times SaO_2 + PaO_2 \times (0.003 \text{ mL } O_2\text{/mm Hg/dL})$$

MORE ON THE DEFINITIONS AND DISTINCTIONS OF PaO_2, SaO_2, AND CaO_2

Unfortunately many people remain confused about the differences among PaO_2, SaO_2, and CaO_2. In the area of blood gas interpretation, this confusion is second only to that surrounding mixed acid–base disorders. Understanding these terms is essential to proper blood gas interpretation; hence the detailed emphasis in this chapter. By the end of this and the next chapter—if you work on all the problems—you should be able to teach the subject!

PaO_2

PaO_2, the partial pressure of oxygen in the plasma phase of arterial blood, is registered by an electrode that senses randomly moving, dissolved oxygen molecules. The amount of dissolved oxygen in the plasma phase—and hence the PaO_2—is determined by alveolar PO_2 and lung architecture only and is unrelated to anything about hemoglobin. (With one exception: When there is both anemia *and* a sizable right-to-left shunt of blood through the lungs, a sufficient amount of blood with low venous O_2 content can enter the arterial circulation and lead to a reduced PaO_2; however, with a normal amount of shunting, anemia and hemoglobin variables *do not* affect PaO_2.)

Oxygen molecules that pass through the thin alveolar–capillary membrane enter the plasma phase as dissolved (free) molecules; most of these molecules quickly enter the red blood cell and bind with hemoglobin (Fig. 5.1). There is a dynamic equilibrium between the freely dissolved and the hemoglobin-bound oxygen molecules. The more dissolved molecules there are (i.e., the greater the PaO_2), the more will bind to the available hemoglobin; thus SaO_2 always depends, to a large degree, on the concentration of dissolved oxygen molecules (i.e., on the PaO_2).

Because there is a virtually unlimited supply of oxygen molecules in the atmosphere, the dissolved O_2 molecules that leave the plasma to bind with hemoglobin are quickly replaced by others; once bound, oxygen no longer exerts a gas pressure. Thus hemoglobin is like an efficient sponge that soaks up oxygen so more can enter the blood. Hemoglobin continues to soak up oxy-

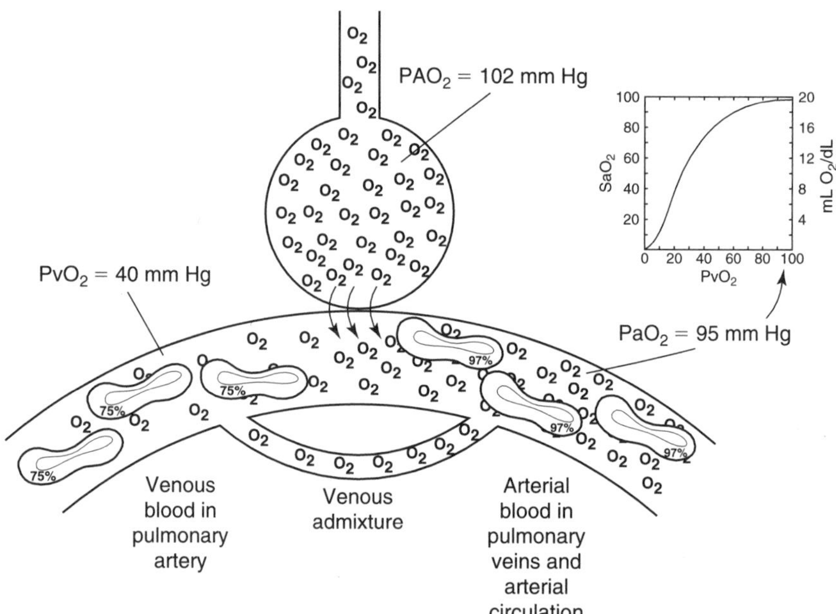

Figure 5.1. Cross section of the lungs and pulmonary circulation, showing oxygen pressure, saturation, and content (CO_2, nitrogen, and other gas molecules are omitted for clarity). PaO_2 is always slightly lower than PAO_2 because of normal venous admixture, here represented by a connection between the venous and pulmonary circulations. Hemoglobin content = 15 g/dL; PAO_2 = 102 mm Hg; PvO_2 = 40 mm Hg; SvO_2 = 75%; PaO_2 = 95 mm Hg; SaO_2 = 97%. See text for discussion.

gen molecules until it becomes saturated with the maximum amount it can hold, which is largely determined by the PaO_2. Of course, this whole process is nearly instantaneous and dynamic; at any given moment a given O_2 molecule could be bound or dissolved. Depending on the PaO_2 and other factors, however, a certain percentage of all O_2 molecules will be dissolved and a certain percentage will be bound (Fig. 5.1). In Figure 5.1, the free or dissolved oxygen molecules register a partial pressure of 95 mm Hg and the red blood cells contain a total hemoglobin content of 15 g/dL.

Each hemoglobin molecule has four Fe^{++}-heme sites for binding oxygen. If there is no interference (as from carbon monoxide, for example), the free O_2 molecules bind to these sites with great avidity. The total percentage of sites actually bound with O_2 is constant for a given set of conditions and is referred to as the *saturation of blood with oxygen.* This is called SvO_2 and SaO_2 in the venous and arterial circulations, respectively; in Figure 5.1, the respective values are 75% and 97%. An SaO_2 of 97% simply means that of every 100 hemoglobin binding sites, 97 are occupied with an oxygen molecule and the other three are either bound to something else or are unbound.

In summary, PaO_2 is determined by alveolar PO_2 and the state of the alveolar–capillary interface, *not* by the amount of hemoglobin available to soak up the oxygen. PaO_2, in turn, determines the oxygen saturation of hemoglobin (along with other factors that affect the position of the O_2 dissociation curve, discussed below). The SaO_2 and the concentration of hemoglobin (15 g/dL in this example) determine the *total* amount of oxygen in the blood, or CaO_2 (see equation for CaO_2). For the variables shown in Figure 5.1, the CaO_2 is 20 mL O_2/dL.

Clinical Problem 5.1. At 10:00 A.M. a patient has a PaO_2 of 85 mm Hg, an SaO_2 of 98%, and a hemoglobin of 14 g/dL. At 10:05 A.M. she suffers a severe hemolytic reaction that suddenly leaves her with a hemoglobin of only 7 g/dL. Assuming no lung disease occurs from the hemolytic reaction, what will be her new PaO_2, SaO_2, and CaO_2?

a. PaO_2 unchanged, SaO_2 unchanged, CaO_2 unchanged
b. PaO_2 unchanged, SaO_2 unchanged, CaO_2 reduced
c. PaO_2 reduced, SaO_2 unchanged, CaO_2 reduced
d. PaO_2 reduced, SaO_2 reduced, CaO_2 reduced

From the forgoing discussion the following observations should now be apparent.

- The less hemoglobin available to bind the dissolved oxygen molecules, the fewer total number of oxygen molecules the blood will contain.
- The more hemoglobin available to bind the dissolved oxygen molecules, the greater total number of oxygen molecules the blood will contain.

Neither the amount of hemoglobin nor the binding characteristics of hemoglobin should affect the amount of *dissolved* oxygen and hence should not affect the PaO_2. Stated another way, the number of dissolved oxygen molecules is *independent* of the amount of hemoglobin or what is bound to it. To repeat one more time (because it is so important), PaO_2 is not a function of hemoglobin content or of its characteristics, but only of the alveolar PO_2 and the lung architecture (alveolar–capillary interface). This explains why, for example, patients with severe anemia or carbon monoxide poisoning or methemoglobinemia can (and often do) have a normal PaO_2.

The most common physiologic disturbance of lung architecture, and hence of a reduced PaO_2, is ventilation–perfusion (V–Q) imbalance. Less common causes are reduced alveolar ventilation, diffusion block, and anatomic right-to-left shunting of blood.

Clinical Problem 5.2 Which of the following situations would be *expected* to lower PaO_2?

a. Anemia
b. Carbon monoxide toxicity
c. An abnormal hemoglobin that holds oxygen with half the affinity of normal hemoglobin
d. An abnormal hemoglobin that holds oxygen with twice the affinity of normal hemoglobin
e. Lung disease with intrapulmonary shunting

SaO_2

SaO_2 is determined mainly by PaO_2. The relationship between the two variables is the familiar oxygen dissociation curve (Fig. 5.2*A*). The dissociation curve is experimentally determined from in vitro titration of blood with increasing partial pressures of oxygen. At low oxygen pressures, there is rela-

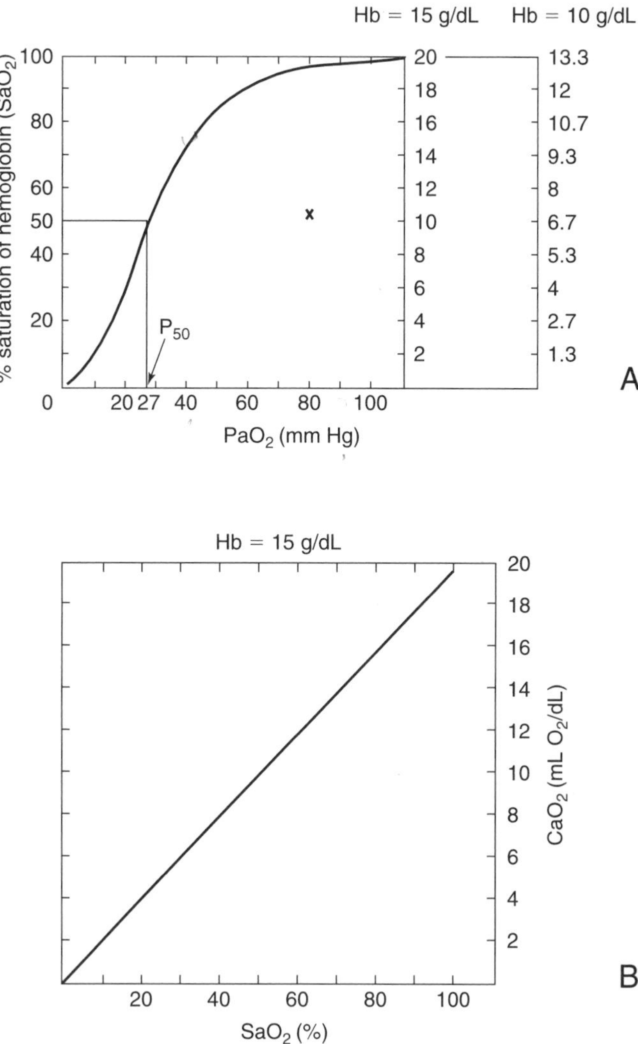

Figure 5.2. A, The oxygen dissociation curve, showing PaO_2 vs. SaO_2 and PaO_2 vs. oxygen content for two different hemoglobin values. P_{50} is the PaO_2 at which hemoglobin is 50% saturated with oxygen; the normal value is 27 mm Hg. *X,* blood gas values of a case presented in Chapter 6. **B,** SaO_2 vs. CaO_2 for a hemoglobin value of 15 g/dL. The relationship between SaO_2 and CaO_2 for any given hemoglobin content is linear (excluding the minor influence of dissolved oxygen with normal PO_2 values).

tively little increase in SaO_2 for a given change in PaO_2. Above a PaO_2 of 20 mm Hg, the rate of change of SaO_2 increases markedly, then slows again beyond a PaO_2 of 60 mm Hg.

PaO_2 is the most important (but not the only) determinant of SaO_2. Other determinants of SaO_2 for a given PaO_2 are conditions that shift the position of the oxygen dissociation curve to the left or right, such as temperature, pH, $PaCO_2$, and 2,3-diphosphoglycerate (2,3-DPG) level in the blood. Shifts of the O_2 dissociation curve will be discussed further in the next chapter.

For now, consolidate your understanding of the difference between PaO_2 and SaO_2. Think of PaO_2 as the driving pressure for oxygen molecules entering the red blood cell and chemically binding to hemoglobin; the higher the PaO_2, the higher the SaO_2. Whatever the SaO_2, its value is simply the percentage of total binding sites on arterial hemoglobin that are bound with oxygen; this value can never be more than 100%.

Clinical Problem 5.3. Using Figure 5.2 to determine SaO_2, calculate the O_2 content of a patient with hemoglobin = 12 g/dL, PaO_2 = 50 mm Hg, and pH = 7.40.

The so-called steep part of the O_2 dissociation curve is between 20 and 60 mm Hg PaO_2. Compared with the flatter portions, small increases in PaO_2 in this region have a much greater effect on improving SaO_2 and, therefore, O_2 content. Figure 5.2*A* shows the oxygen dissociation curve for PaO_2 plotted against the oxygen content for two hemoglobin concentrations: 15 and 10 g/dL. Note that the *shape and position* of the curve are the same irrespective of the hemoglobin content.

SaO_2 is unaffected by the hemoglobin content, so anemia does not lower SaO_2. The more hemoglobin, the more oxygen molecules will be bound in a given volume of blood. The *percentage* of available hemoglobin sites bound to oxygen (the SaO_2) depends only on the PaO_2 and curve-shifting factors. Thus a patient can have normal PaO_2 and SaO_2 but still have a low CaO_2 (e.g., with anemia).

CaO_2

CaO_2, unlike either PaO_2 or SaO_2, directly reflects the total number of oxygen molecules in arterial blood, both bound and unbound to hemoglobin. In contrast to the other two variables, CaO_2 depends on the hemoglobin content and is directly related to it; other determinants of CaO_2 are the SaO_2 (which depends on PaO_2 and the position of the oxygen dissociation curve) and the amount of dissolved oxygen (the PaO_2). Because the dissolved oxygen contributes minimally to CaO_2 under physiologic conditions, CaO_2 is determined almost entirely by hemoglobin content and SaO_2 and is related linearly to either variable (Fig. 5.2*B*).

Normal CaO_2 ranges from 16 to 22 mL O_2/dL. Because PaO_2 and/or SaO_2 can be normal in certain conditions associated with hypoxemia, one should always make sure CaO_2 is adequate when assessing oxygenation. About 98% of the normal O_2 content is carried bound to hemoglobin.

The CaO_2 component bound to hemoglobin can be calculated by

$$Hb \times 1.34 \times SaO_2$$

and the dissolved component by

$$0.003 \times PaO_2$$

The CaO_2 equation (see Chapter 2) be used to calculate the oxygen content of any blood or plasma sample.

Figure 5.3 shows two beakers containing liquid open to the atmosphere. Beaker 1 contains blood with a Hb content of 15 g/dL. Beaker 2 contains only plasma (no hemoglobin). Assuming a barometric pressure of 760 mm Hg (and no water vapor pressure), calculate the oxygen content in each beaker.

Beaker 1 contains hemoglobin that will combine chemically with oxygen; hence the oxygen content in beaker 1 consists of bound and unbound (dissolved) oxygen molecules. In beaker 2 there is no hemoglobin, just pure plasma; all of its oxygen content must come from dissolved oxygen.

Dissolved oxygen in both beakers is determined by the PO_2 to which the liquid is exposed and the solubility of oxygen in plasma. The solubility is 0.003 mL O_2/dL plasma/mm Hg. But what is the PO_2? Because there is no CO_2 exchange taking place in either beaker (as there is in our lungs) and the surface of the liquid is in free contact with the atmosphere, the PO_2 *in* the solution is simply the PO_2 *above* the solution. Given a barometric pressure of 760 mm Hg (dry air), the PO_2 in both beakers is

$$FIO_2 \times P_B = 0.21 \times 760 \text{ mm Hg} = 160 \text{ mm Hg}$$

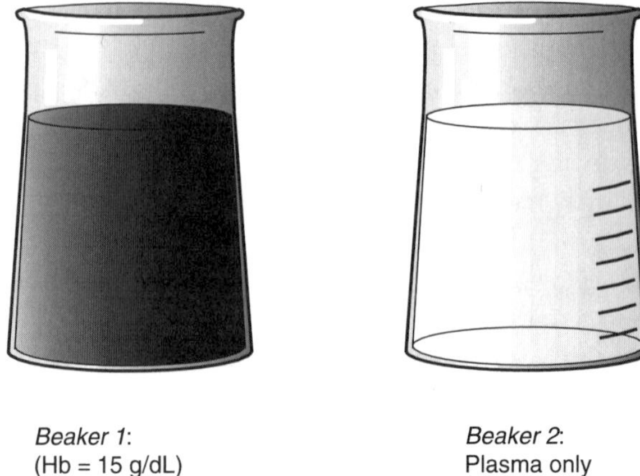

Figure 5.3. Beaker 1 contains blood with a hemoglobin content of 15 g/dL; beaker 2 contains pure plasma (no hemoglobin). Both beakers are open to the atmosphere (dry air; barometric pressure = 760 mm Hg).

Since the PO_2 is equal in both beakers, the O_2 content represented by *dissolved oxygen* is also the same in both beakers; this content is

a. 0.48 mL O_2/dL
b. 2.0 mL O_2/dL
c. 4.8 mL O_2/dL

To calculate content from dissolved oxygen, substitute the values for oxygen solubility and PO_2:

$$O_2 \text{ content from dissolved } O_2 = 0.003 \text{ mL } O_2/\text{dL/mm Hg} \times 160 \text{ mm Hg} = 0.48 \text{ mL } O_2/\text{dL}$$

There is no hemoglobin in beaker 2 so the *entirety* of its O_2 content comes from dissolved oxygen and thus is equal to 0.48 mL O_2/dL. There is far more oxygen content in beaker 1 because oxygen molecules combine chemically with hemoglobin. Once combined, O_2 molecules no longer exert any pressure. As O_2 molecules are taken up by hemoglobin, additional molecules enter the plasma portion of the blood from the atmosphere. Remember: **Hemoglobin is like a sponge that soaks up free oxygen molecules and allows many more to enter the surrounding plasma.**

Thus the difference in oxygen content between the two beakers is the amount of oxygen bound to the hemoglobin.

The oxygen content represented by *hemoglobin-bound* oxygen in beaker 1 is

a. 0.48 mL O_2/dL
b. 15 mL O_2/dL
c. 19.9 mL O_2/dL

The O_2 content is calculated by the oxygen content equation, which in turn requires knowledge of SaO_2, the saturation of hemoglobin with oxygen. SaO_2 is determined by the PO_2 to which the blood is exposed in the lungs (in this case 160 mm Hg) *and* the position of the oxygen dissociation curve. With a normally positioned curve, the SaO_2 at this level of PO_2 is approximately 99%. Thus

$$\begin{aligned}\text{Oxygen content (Hb-bound)} &= \text{Hb} \times 1.34 \times SaO_2 \\ &= 15 \times 1.34 \times 0.99 \\ &= 19.9 \text{ mL } O_2/\text{dL}\end{aligned}$$

What is the *total* oxygen content of beaker 1? By what factor is this content greater than that in beaker 2?

The total oxygen content of beaker 1 is, of course, the sum of the dissolved and bound fractions, or 0.48 + 19.9 = 20.38 mL O_2/dL. The total oxygen content of beaker 2 (0.48 mL O_2/dL) is thus only about 2.4% of that contained in beaker 1. Put another way, beaker 1 contains about 42 times more oxygen than beaker 2.

Clinical Problem 5.4. A healthy man is in the same room as the two beakers shown in Figure 5.3. If his PaO_2 = 100 mm Hg and Hb content = 15 g/dL, what percent of his oxygen content is carried in dissolved form?

To summarize much of the forgoing discussion:

- Although almost all of the oxygen content is chemically bound to hemoglobin, this quantity is unrevealed by knowing only the PaO_2.
- Without knowledge of the hemoglobin content, the PaO_2 does not even give a hint of the total oxygen content.
- We need to calculate CaO_2 to know the *amount* of oxygen in the blood.
- Because the body needs a specific oxygen content for survival, and PaO_2 alone does not indicate oxygen content, *a patient can have normal PaO_2 and be starved for oxygen.*

Clinical Problem 5.5. For each of the four situations below, give the expected changes (increased, decreased, or normal) for PaO_2, SaO_2, and CaO_2. Assume the subject is breathing ambient air, that each situation occurred acutely (in < 24 h), and that there is no other abnormal condition.

Measure	Severe anemia	CO Poisoning	Severe V–Q imbalance	High altitude
PaO_2				
SaO_2				
CaO_2				

Clinical Problem 5.6. Which patient is more hypoxemic?

Patient A: $PaO_2 = 85$ mm Hg, $SaO_2 = 95\%$, Hb $= 7$ g/dL
Patient B: $PaO_2 = 55$ mm Hg, $SaO_2 = 85\%$, Hb $= 15$ g/dL

Clinical Problem 5.7. Test your understanding by indicating whether the following statements are true or false. If you understand the material in this chapter you should get all of them right.

a. If the lungs and heart are normal, then PaO_2 is affected only by the alveolar PO_2.

b. In a person with normal heart and lungs, anemia should not lower the PaO_2.
c. PaO_2 will go up in a patient with hemolysis of red blood cells, as dissolved oxygen is given off when the cells lyse.
d. As the oxygen dissociation curve shifts to the right, PaO_2 rises since less oxygen is bound to hemoglobin.
e. An anemic patient who receives a blood transfusion should experience a rise in both SaO_2 and CaO_2.
f. The PaO_2 in a cup of water is zero since there is no blood perfusing the water.
g. The SaO_2 in a cup of water is zero since there is no hemoglobin present.
h. The CaO_2 in a cup of water is zero since there is no hemoglobin present.

HYPOXEMIA VS. HYPOXIA

Clinical Problem 5.6 asks which patient is more hypoxemic, and the answer is found by calculating the oxygen contents. Would the answer have been different if the question were, "Which patient is more *hypoxic*?" What is the difference between *hypoxemia* and *hypoxia* and does it matter? Some textbooks use the words interchangeably, whereas others define them differently.

There is no universal agreement on the terms, and the distinction is partly semantic. I prefer to define hypoxemia as a reduction in PaO_2, SaO_2, *or* hemoglobin content (Table 5.1); the *amount* of oxygen in the blood (oxygen content) is the major determinant of severity. In this context, the lower the oxygen content, the more hypoxemic the patient, irrespective of the PaO_2 or SaO_2.

Hypoxia, on the other hand, is a more general term referring to impaired oxygen delivery to the tissues. Hypoxia takes into account cardiac output and oxygen uptake at the tissue level. In this scheme, hypoxemia is but one type of hypoxia (Table 5.1). A patient can have hypoxemia but still maintain adequate O_2 delivery to the tissues, through adaptive increases in cardiac output and/or O_2 extraction at the tissue level; in that situation, the hypoxemic patient will not be hypoxic. Conversely, a patient can have an adequate oxygen content but be hypoxic, as may occur in a low cardiac output state or from mitochondrial poisoning.

TABLE 5.1. CAUSES OF HYPOXIA—A GENERAL CLASSIFICATION

1. Hypoxemia
   a. Reduced PaO_2 (see Table 4.3)
   b. Reduced SaO_2 (any cause of 1a; carbon monoxide poisoning; excess methemoglobin; and any cause of a right-shifted oxygen dissociation curve, such as acidemia)
   c. Reduced hemoglobin content (anemia)
2. Reduced oxygen delivery to the tissues
   a. Reduced cardiac output (shock, congestive heart failure)
   b. Left-to-right systemic shunt (as may be seen in septic shock)
3. Decreased tissue oxygen uptake
   a. Mitochondrial poisoning (cyanide poisoning)
   b. Left-shifted hemoglobin dissociation curve (alkalemia, carbon monoxide poisoning, abnormal hemoglobin structure)

In the final analysis, it doesn't really matter how the terms are used as long as you understand the differences between oxygen pressure, saturation, and content. Understand these concepts, and you can define hypoxemia and hypoxia any way you wish.

CLINICAL ASSESSMENT OF HYPOXEMIA

Before the era of rapid blood gas analysis, clinicians would often assess hypoxemia on clinical grounds alone, principally by looking for cyanosis. We now know that clinical assessment of hypoxemia is unreliable (notoriously so), for several reasons:

- There is significant interobserver variation in detecting cyanosis; some physicians diagnose cyanosis when it cannot be present (normal blood gases) and some miss cyanosis when it is present (very low oxygen saturation) (Comroe & Botelho 1947).
- It takes approximately 5 g/dL of unoxygenated hemoglobin in the capillaries to generate the dark blue color appreciated clinically as cyanosis (Lundsgaard & Van Slyke 1923, Martin & Khalil 1990). Anemic patients may be significantly hypoxemic yet be unable to generate this much reduced hemoglobin. A severely anemic patient whose hemoglobin content is only 5 g/dL (giving a hematocrit about 15%) would never manifest cyanosis no matter how hypoxemic.
- Ancillary signs and symptoms of hypoxemia (tachycardia, tachypnea, mental status changes) are not specific enough to be of value in reliably detect-

ing hypoxemia. Patients may be profoundly dyspneic with normal PaO_2 and SaO_2. Also, some patients who are profoundly hypoxemic may remain lucid and fully conversant.

If you have any reason to suspect hypoxemia, obtain some measurement of the oxygen level (arterial blood gas or pulse oximetry). There is no clinical substitute for measurement of PaO_2 or SaO_2 when diagnosing hypoxemia or assessing the need for supplemental oxygen therapy.

ANSWERS TO CLINICAL PROBLEMS

5.1. b. PaO_2 unchanged, SaO_2 unchanged, CaO_2 reduced. Hemoglobin content is suddenly reduced by half, which will lower CaO_2 by half; however, the PaO_2 and SaO_2 will be unaffected, because their values are independent of the content of hemoglobin present.

5.2. Of the choices given only answer e, lung disease with intrapulmonary shunting, would be expected to lower PaO_2. The other choices represent changes in hemoglobin content and binding and should not (by themselves) lower PaO_2.

5.3. To calculate oxygen content, you first need to find the SaO_2. From Figure 5.3, you can see that SaO_2 is about 83% (in using the graph ±1% is acceptable). Ignoring the dissolved oxygen fraction (which is very small), the O_2 content is

$$CaO_2 = 0.83 \times 12 \times 1.34 = 13.35 \text{ mL } O_2/\text{dL}$$

Note that this content falls midway between the oxygen content values for hemoglobin of 10 and 15 g/dL.

5.4. The calculation is the same as with the two beakers, except that PO_2 is 100 mm Hg instead of 160 mm Hg (PO_2 is lower than atmospheric pressure because of the addition of water vapor pressure and $PaCO_2$); thus his dissolved fraction is 0.3 mL O_2/dL instead of 0.48 mL O_2/dL in the beakers. His O_2-bound fraction is also slightly lower, because a PO_2 of 100 mm Hg gives an SaO_2 of about 98%. Thus the oxygen content in human blood under these conditions is

$$\begin{aligned} CaO_2 &= (\text{Hb} \times 1.34 \times SaO_2) + (0.003 \times PaO_2) \\ &= (15 \times 1.34 \times 0.98) + (0.003 \times 100) \\ &= 19.7 + 0.3 \\ &= 20.0 \text{ mL } O_2/\text{dL} \end{aligned}$$

The dissolved O_2 content is 0.3/20 = 1.5% of the total oxygen content. Stated another way, under these conditions (normal PaO_2 and hemoglobin content), hemoglobin carries about *67 times more* oxygen than is carried dissolved in the plasma. Clearly, hemoglobin is vital. Under conditions of ambient air and pressure, the content of dissolved oxygen is far too little to meet our metabolic needs.

5.5.

Measure	Severe anemia	CO poisoning	Severe V–Q imbalance	High altitude
PaO_2	Normal	Normal	Decreased	Decreased
SaO_2	Normal	Decreased	Decreased	Decreased
CaO_2	Decreased	Decreased	Decreased	Decreased

5.6. The body needs oxygen molecules, so oxygen content (CaO_2) takes precedence over partial pressure in determining degrees of hypoxemia. In this problem, the amount of oxygen contributed by the dissolved fraction is negligible and will not affect the answer.

Patient A: $CaO_2 = 0.95 \times 7 \times 1.34 = 8.9$ mL O_2/dL
Patient B: $CaO_2 = 0.85 \times 15 \times 1.34 = 17.1$ mL O_2/dL

Patient A, with the higher PaO_2, is more hypoxemic.

5.7

a. True
b. True
c. False
d. False
e. False
f. False
g. True
h. False

CHAPTER

6

SaO_2, Hemoglobin Binding, and Pulse Oximetry

OXYGENATED AND REDUCED HEMOGLOBIN

Chapter 5 emphasized important distinctions between PaO_2, SaO_2, and CaO_2. This chapter will expand on that topic with discussions of hemoglobin binding, carboxyhemoglobin, methemoglobin, and pulse oximetry.

First, some clarification of terminology. Although the terms *hypoxemia* and *hypoxia* tend to be user defined, other oxygen-related terms are more rigorously defined yet are often just as confusing (if not more so). Consider the following blood gas values in a patient breathing room air:

pH	7.42
$PaCO_2$	34 mm Hg
PaO_2	67 mm Hg
SaO_2	84%
COHb	5%
MetHb	2%

What are the approximate percentages for each of the following in this patient's blood?

Oxygenated hemoglobin ____________________
Reduced hemoglobin ____________________
Deoxygenated hemoglobin ____________________
Oxidized hemoglobin ____________________
Carboxyhemoglobin ____________________
Methemoglobin ____________________

Oxygenated hemoglobin refers to heme groups bound with oxygen. It is quantified by the SaO_2, which expresses the percentage of all the heme groups bound with O_2. *Reduced hemoglobin* is another term for *deoxygenated* hemoglobin and refers to all the heme groups unbound to oxygen or to anything else. (Strictly speaking, the terms should be "oxygenated heme" and "unoxygenated heme," because *a single* hemoglobin molecule—with four heme binding sites—could contain *both* oxygenated and unoxygenated heme moieties.)

For the above blood gas data, the percentage of oxygenated hemoglobin is the same as the measured SaO_2, i.e., 84%. The percentage of deoxygenated (reduced) hemoglobin is found by subtracting all the hemoglobin either bound to something (SaO_2 and COHb) or that cannot bind oxygen (MetHb); thus the percentage of deoxygenated hemoglobin is 9%.

Maximum oxygen saturation	100%
SaO_2	84%
COHb	5%
MetHb	2%
Deoxygenated (reduced) Hb	9%

Oxidized hemoglobin is hemoglobin with iron in an oxidized state (Fe^{+++}) as opposed to the normal ferrous (Fe^{++}) state; hemoglobin with Fe^{+++} is called *methemoglobin,* which, in this example, makes up 2% of the total. Note that even though Fe^{+++} hemoglobin is oxidized, the normal Fe^{++} state of hemoglobin is *not* called "reduced"; reduced hemoglobin refers only to Fe^{++} hemoglobin that is not bound with oxygen or anything else. The terminology is perhaps confusing and unfortunate; however, because it is widely used, you should familiarize yourself with the generally accepted definitions.

Carboxyhemoglobin, already defined, makes up 5% of the total hemoglobin in the above example, a slightly elevated value.

THE IMPORTANCE OF MEASURING (AND NOT JUST CALCULATING) SaO_2

PaO_2 is a measurement of the partial pressure exerted by oxygen molecules dissolved in plasma. Once oxygen molecules chemically bind to hemoglobin they no longer exert any pressure. Patients can have a low PaO_2 (most commonly from a V–Q imbalance) and still have adequate arterial oxygen content, e.g., hemoglobin = 15 g/dL, PaO_2 = 55 mm Hg, SaO_2 = 88%, and CaO_2 =

17.8 mL O_2/dL blood. Conversely, as was discussed in Chapter 5, patients can have a normal PaO_2 and be *profoundly hypoxemic* from reduced CaO_2. This paradox—normal PaO_2 and hypoxemia—generally occurs two ways: anemia or altered affinity of hemoglobin for binding oxygen.

CASE. *A 54-year-old man came to the emergency room (ER) complaining of headaches and dyspnea. An arterial blood gas (on room air) showed PaO_2 = 89 mm Hg, $PaCO_2$ = 38 mm Hg, and pH = 7.43. SaO_2 was not directly measured but was calculated at 98% based on the measured PaO_2 and a standard oxygen dissociation curve. His hemoglobin content was normal at 14.6 g/dL. He was sent home after some improvement in the ER and was scheduled for a brain CT scan two days later.*

The next evening he was brought back to the ER unconscious. Ambulance attendants alerted the emergency physicians to a possible faulty heater in the patient's house. This time carbon monoxide and SaO_2 were measured directly with a co-oximeter, along with arterial blood gases. The results: PaO_2 = 79 mm Hg, $PaCO_2$ = 31 mm Hg, pH = 7.36, SaO_2 = 53%, carboxyhemoglobin = 46%.

What do you suppose was the patient's true SaO_2 on the initial ER visit?

a. Probably > 90%
b. Probably < 90%
c. Don't know how to guess the answer

The true SaO_2 was much lower than 90%, as would have been apparent had it been measured on the initial ER visit, instead of just calculated. Generally, a patient needs at least 10% COHb to manifest symptoms from excess CO (Table 6.1). The first blood gas did not pick up the CO poisoning because, as was pointed out in Chapter 5, carbon monoxide per se does not affect PaO_2, but only SaO_2 and O_2 content. (The PaO_2 was slightly lower on the return ER visit owing to some basilar atelectasis that had developed.) The patient's oxygen saturation and content on the return visit are shown by the *X* in Figure 5.2.

This case illustrates the importance of *measuring* the SaO_2 as part of each arterial blood gas test. A *calculated* SaO_2 (as shown above) can be misleading.

TABLE 6.1. SYMPTOMS OF CO POISONING

CO IN INSPIRED AIR, %	COHb IN BLOOD, %	OCCURRENCE; SIGNS AND SYMPTOMS
0	1–2	Normal amount from breakdown of heme; no symptoms
< 0.007	3–10	Common in cigarette smokers; no symptoms, but may aggravate dyspnea from other causes
0.007	> 10	Found in heavy cigarette and cigar smokers; dyspnea during vigorous exertion, occasional tightness in forehead
0.012	> 20	Dyspnea during moderate exertion; occasional throbbing headache in temples
0.022	> 30	Severe headache, irritability, easily fatigued, disturbed judgment, possible dizziness, possible dimness of vision
0.035–0.052	> 40	Headache, confusion, syncope with exertion
0.080–0.122	> 60	Unconsciousness, shock, intermittent convulsions, respiratory failure, death if exposure is prolonged
0.195	> 70	Death

The physician on the first visit missed hypoxemia as a cause of headache and dyspnea because of the falsely "normal" SaO_2.

P_{50} AND SHIFTS OF THE OXYGEN DISSOCIATION CURVE

Many factors can affect the degree of oxygen saturation for a given PaO_2; their net result is the exact shape and position of the oxygen dissociation curve.

From the following list choose those factors that affect the binding of oxygen to hemoglobin for a given PaO_2.

a. Age of the patient
b. PAO_2
c. $PaCO_2$
d. pH

e. Carbon monoxide
f. Nature of the hemoglobin molecule
g. Body temperature
h. 2,3-diphosphoglycerate (2,3-DPG) in blood
i. Hemoglobin content

The shape and position of the oxygen dissociation curve are affected by all of the factors listed above except the age of the patient, PAO_2, and hemoglobin content. What about these exceptions?

- Characteristics of the whole patient (age, body weight, body position, etc.) can affect the PaO_2 by altering ventilation–perfusion relationships (Chapter 4) but have no direct effect on how oxygen binds with hemoglobin.
- Although PAO_2 is a major determinant of PaO_2 (Chapter 4), it has no effect on the binding of oxygen to hemoglobin (i.e., on the SaO_2).
- A common misconception is that anemia somehow changes the binding of oxygen to hemoglobin. In fact, anemia does not affect the position of the O_2 dissociation curve. Stated another way, the amount of hemoglobin affects the O_2 content but not the extent to which oxygen binds to the available hemoglobin.

All the other listed factors can affect the degree of O_2 binding to hemoglobin for a given PaO_2. Figure 6.1 separates these factors according to how they shift the oxygen dissociation curve. Figure 6.2 shows specific curve shifts with changes in pH and temperature.

A shift of the O_2 dissociation curve to the right means:

a. Less SaO_2 for a given PaO_2
b. More SaO_2 for a given PaO_2

If a PaO_2 of 60 mm Hg normally gives an SaO_2 of 90%, and the oxygen dissociation curve is shifted to the right, the same PaO_2 will give a lower SaO_2. The correct answer is therefore a.

Clinical Problem 6.1. For the following paired samples, state whether patient 1 or 2 has the lower arterial oxygen content (i.e., which patient is more hypoxemic?). When necessary, use Figure 6.2 to determine approximate SaO_2 values.

a.
Patient 1: Hb = 10 g/dL, PaO_2 = 60 mm Hg, pH = 7.55
Patient 2: Hb = 10 g/dL, PaO_2 = 60 mm Hg, pH = 7.35
b.
Patient 1: Hb = 15 g/dL, PaO_2 = 90 mm Hg, pH = 7.10
Patient 2: Hb = 15 g/dL, PaO_2 = 60 mm Hg, pH = 7.47
c.
Patient 1: Hb = 12 g/dL, SaO_2 = 90%, pH = 7.20
Patient 2: Hb = 12 g/dL, SaO_2 = 80%, pH = 7.40
d.
Patient 1: Hb = 12 g/dL, PaO_2 = 90 mm Hg, pH = 7.40
Patient 2: Hb = 12 g/dL, SaO_2 = 90%, pH = 7.40

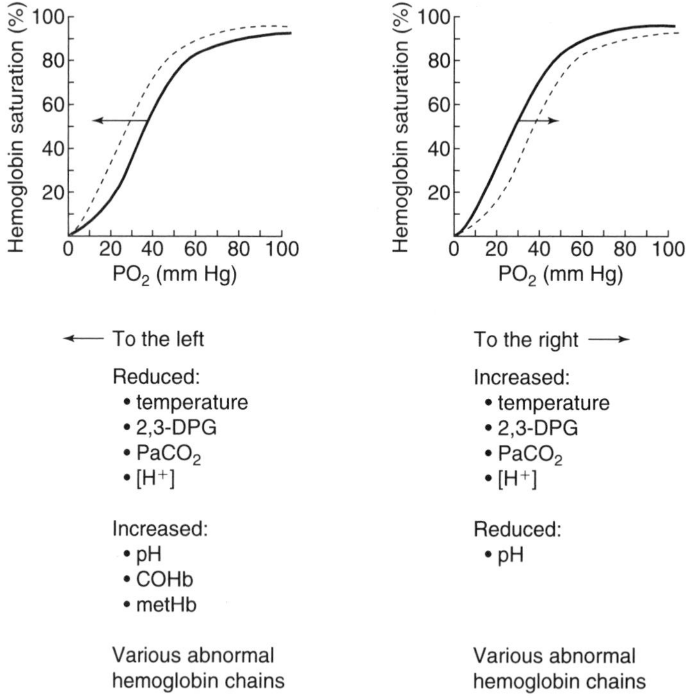

Figure 6.1. Conditions that can shift the oxygen dissociation curve.

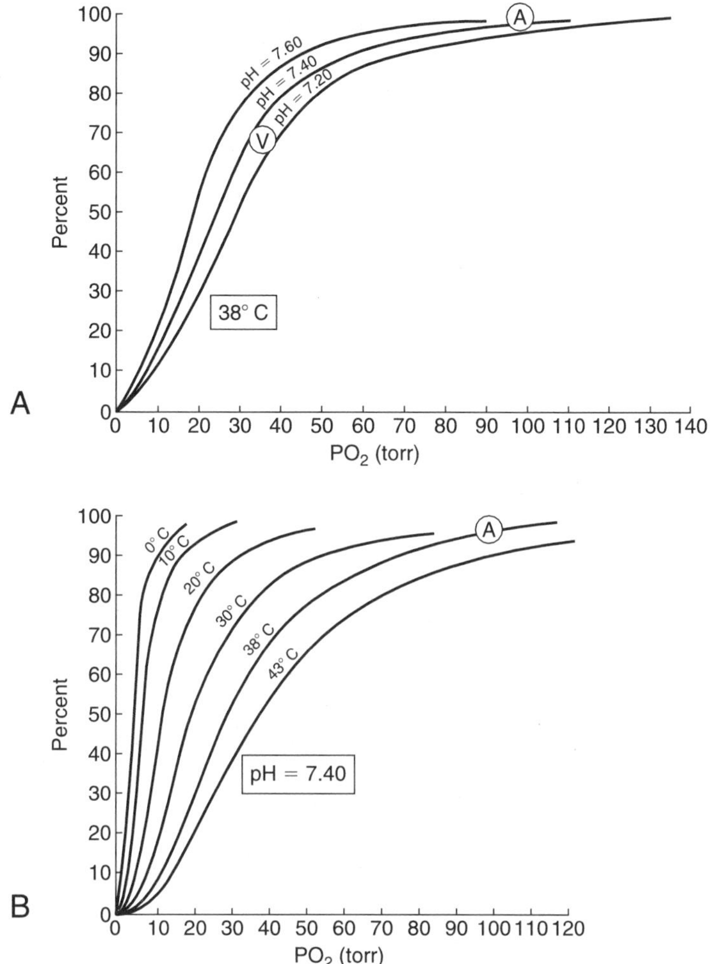

Figure 6.2. Shifts of the O_2 dissociation curve with (**A**) changes in pH (temperature constant) and (**B**) changes in temperature (pH constant). Modified from Slonim NB, Hamilton LH. Respiratory physiology. 4th ed. St. Louis: Mosby, 1981.

P_{50} is the PaO_2 at which 50% of the arterial hemoglobin is saturated with oxygen, i.e., the PaO_2 at which $SaO_2 = 50\%$. P_{50} is a time-consuming and non-routine measurement, performed only in some blood gas labs on special request. It is used to characterize the degree of shift of the oxygen dissociation curve. Normal P_{50} is about 27 mm Hg.

A rightward shift of the dissociation curve would manifest as:

a. $P_{50} > 27$ mm Hg
b. $P_{50} < 27$ mm Hg

In which direction is the O_2 dissociation curve shifted if P_{50} is 24 mm Hg?

a. To the right
b. To the left

Examination of the oxygen dissociation curve shows that a higher than normal P_{50} reflects a rightward shift of the curve and a lower than normal P_{50}, a leftward shift (remember the mnemonic *low* P_{50} = *leftward shift*).

Clinical Problem 6.2. Fill in the P_{50} column by placing the correct value for the given pH and PCO_2 values. Choose among the following values for P_{50}: 22, 24.5, 27, 29.5, and 31 mm Hg.

pH	PCO_2	P_{50}
7.26	60	
7.32	50	
7.40	40	
7.48	30	
7.56	20	

Generally, a left-shifted curve results in holding back more oxygen at the tissue level than is gained in the pulmonary capillaries; this results in a higher SaO_2, while, paradoxically, less oxygen is delivered to the tissues. When the curve is shifted to the right, the opposite occurs; less oxygen is taken up in the pulmonary capillaries but relatively more is unloaded at the tissue level.

What is better for the hypoxemic patient: a left shift or right shift of the oxygen dissociation curve? Should therapy be directed toward artificially shifting the curve one way or the other? Before answering these questions, review Figure 6.2.

Some people argue that a right-shifted curve is better for the critically ill patient than even a normal dissociation curve, since more oxygen is unloaded at the tissues. The metabolic acidosis that invariably accompanies a shock state could be nature's way of ensuring that more oxygen is delivered to the tissues.

Unfortunately, this physiologic argument doesn't translate into clinical strategy. While a right-shifted curve unloads more oxygen to the tissues, if the shift occurs at the cost of acidemia, high $PaCO_2$, or fever, the patient might suffer in other ways. The best clinical answer to this question is that *neither* shift is necessarily better. One should aim for an adequate oxygen content and cardiac output and not attempt to manipulate the oxygen dissociation curve.

CARBOXYHEMOGLOBIN AND THE O_2 DISSOCIATION CURVE

Figure 6.3 shows how elevated carbon monoxide affects the oxygen dissociation curve. Carbon monoxide affects tissue oxygen delivery in two ways: It reduces arterial oxygen saturation by preventing oxygen binding to hemoglobin; and it increases affinity for those oxygen molecules that do bind to hemoglobin, i.e., it causes a left shift of the oxygen dissociation curve (Ernst 1998).

Carbon monoxide is about 230 times more avid for hemoglobin than is oxygen. Thus a partial pressure of CO at only 1/230 of that of oxygen will compete equally for hemoglobin binding sites. If PaO_2 is 100 mm Hg and PaCO is only 0.43 mm Hg, the blood will contain 50% oxyhemoglobin and 50% COHb. Obviously, it only takes tiny amounts of CO to induce poisoning.

Figure 6.3 shows the double-whammy effect of excess CO on oxygenation. First, to the extent that CO is bound to hemoglobin, oxygen is prevented from binding to those same sites. Binding of oxygen and CO takes place in the pulmonary capillaries as the gases are inhaled. If enough CO is inhaled to bind with 30% of the hemoglobin (30% COHb), for example, then 30% of the hemoglobin binding sites are effectively prevented from combining with oxygen. The maximum that SaO_2 could ever reach would be 70%, irrespective of the PaO_2.

Second, CO increases the affinity of hemoglobin for oxygen molecules that *are* chemically bound. Increased affinity means hemoglobin holds on to oxygen

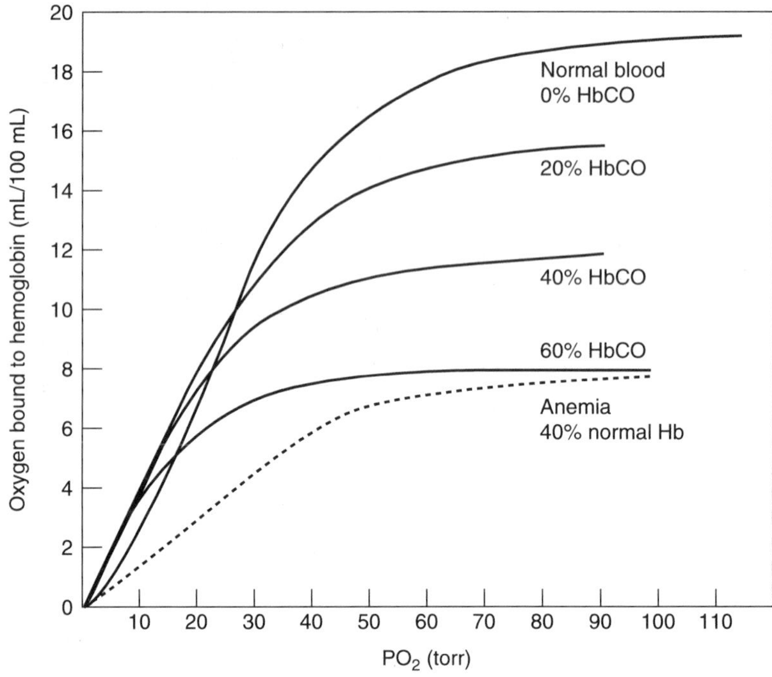

Figure 6.3. Effects of carbon monoxide on the oxygen dissociation curve. See text for discussion. Modified from Roughton FJW, Darling RC. Am J Physiol 1944;141:17–31 and reprinted with permission from Comroe JH Jr. Physiology of respiration. 2nd ed. Chicago: Year Book Medical Publishers, 1974.

molecules *more tightly* in the presence of excess CO; as a result, the oxygen dissociation curve is shifted to the *left.* The adverse effect of this left shift is greatest at the tissue capillary level, as can be seen in Figure 6.3. At PO_2 values found in the tissue capillaries (20–40 mm Hg), oxygen is bound more tightly to the hemoglobin, i.e., less is given up to the tissues.

In the pulmonary capillary, severe anemia (40% of the normal hemoglobin content) has about the same effect on O_2 content as 60% COHb (Fig. 6.3); however, a big difference emerges at the tissue level. When the blood circulates to the tissues, the anemic blood unloads oxygen much more readily than the blood with excess CO. Thus for PO_2 values at the tissue level (e.g., 30 mm Hg), the oxygen saturation (and content) are much higher in the presence of excess CO. The patient with excess CO is thus more *hypoxic* than the patient with anemia, because CO-laden hemoglobin holds on to oxygen much more strongly.

In summary, excess CO causes

- Less oxygen to bind to hemoglobin in the pulmonary capillaries.
- Oxygen that is taken up by hemoglobin to be held more tightly than normal, making less oxygen available to the tissues for any given PO_2 value.

These two effects, plus its very high affinity for hemoglobin, make CO a potent poison.

Clinical Problem 6.3. Below are blood gas results from four pairs of patients. For each pair, state which patient, 1 or 2, is more hypoxemic.

a.
Patient 1: Hb = 15 g/dL, PaO_2 = 100 mm Hg, pH = 7.40, COHb = 20%
Patient 2: Hb = 12 g/dL, PaO_2 = 100 mm Hg, pH = 7.40, COHb = 0%

b.
Patient 1: Hb = 15 g/dL, PaO_2 = 90 mm Hg, pH = 7.20, COHb = 5%
Patient 2: Hb = 15 g/dL, PaO_2 = 50 mm Hg, pH = 7.40, COHb = 0%

c.
Patient 1: Hb = 5 g/dL, PaO_2 = 60 mm Hg, pH = 7.40, COHb = 0%
Patient 2: Hb = 15 g/dL, PaO_2 = 100 mm Hg, pH = 7.40, COHb = 20%

d.
Patient 1: Hb = 10 g/dL, PaO_2 = 60 mm Hg, pH = 7.30, COHb = 10%
Patient 2: Hb = 15 g/dL, PaO_2 = 100 mm Hg, pH = 7.40, COHb = 15%

Carbon monoxide is competitively bound to hemoglobin and, therefore, easily removable if the PO_2 is high enough. Treatment of CO poisoning requires elevating PaO_2 as quickly as possible, the higher the better. In most cases, this is accomplished with an FIO_2 equal or close to 100%, for at least the first few hours of therapy. Extreme cases of CO poisoning (presenting with coma or convulsions) require intubation and mechanical ventilation with 100% oxygen. In hospitals with a hyperbaric chamber, oxygen can be delivered under increased pressures (e.g., two to three times normal atmospheric pressure), effecting an even quicker removal of excess CO. The goal in all cases is to "flush out" the CO as quickly as possible with supplemental oxygen.

PULSE OXIMETRY

Noninvasive measurement of hemoglobin-oxygen saturation has been possible for decades, but only since the late 1980s has it become both widely available and easily performed. The change took place with the advent of small and reliable machines that can sense a patient's pulse (usually in a digit) and, by emitting two wavelengths of light, differentiate oxygenated from deoxygenated hemoglobin (Clark et al. 1992; Leasa 1992; Schnapp & Cohen 1990). A pulse oximeter with its reading is shown in Figure 6.4.

Because the oxygen saturation measured by pulse oximetry is not the same as the SaO_2 measured by CO oximetry on arterial blood, the term *SpO_2* is used to indicate the pulse oximeter value. Understanding the differences between SaO_2 and SpO_2 should help you avoid pitfalls when using the pulse oximeter. These differences are listed in Table 6.2 and discussed below.

Note that the differences between SpO_2-measured and co-oximetry-measured SaO_2 are based mainly on available technology. Although the technology continues to evolve, current pulse oximeters use only *two* wavelengths of light sent noninvasively through a finger (or toe or earlobe), whereas co-oximeters send *four* wavelengths of light through a blood sample. Four wavelengths (but not two) allows differentiation of oxyhemoglobin from carboxyhemoglobin and

TABLE 6.2. CO-OXIMETRY VS. PULSE OXIMETRY

CHARACTERISTIC	CO-OXIMETER	PULSE OXIMETER
Number of wavelengths of light	4	2
Technique	In vitro; arterial blood sample inserted into the machine (Fig. 1.1)	Noninvasive: digit or earlobe, where a pulse can be sensed easily by a portable machine (Fig. 6.4)
Measures	$\%O_2Hb$ (SaO_2); % unbound Hb; %COHb; %MetHb; Hb content	$\%O_2Hb$ (SaO_2); % unbound Hb
Advantages	Highly accurate; can distinguish COHb from O_2Hb	Painless; allows for continuous monitoring; easily portable; relatively inexpensive; SpO_2 not affected by fetal Hb
Major disadvantages	Requires arterial sample; expensive to purchase, maintain, and operate; not available for most outpatients; fetal Hb interferes with SaO_2 reading	Doesn't differentiate COHb from O_2Hb; may give false sense of security in setting of progressive hypercapnia with supplemental O_2; correlation of SpO_2 with SaO_2 varies among machines; can be misused by caregivers unfamiliar with basic principles

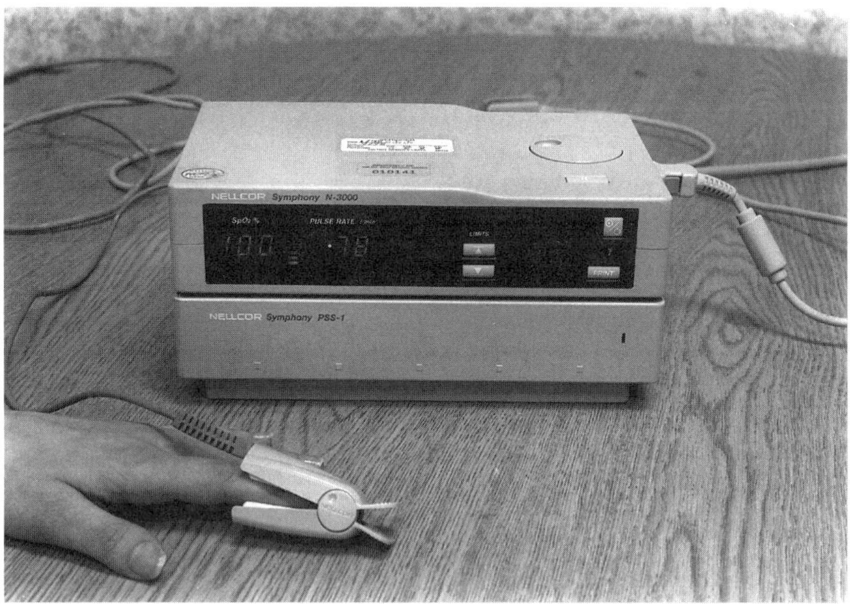

Figure 6.4. Finger pulse oximeter with reading. The subject's pulse rate is 78/min and SpO_2 is 100%.

TABLE 6.3. HOW SOME FACTORS INFLUENCE PULSE OXIMETRY READING OF OXYGEN SATURATION[a]

FACTOR	SpO_2 READING IS
Carboxyhemoglobin	Higher than true SaO_2
Methemoglobin	Higher than true SaO_2
Dark nail polish	Slightly lower than true SaO_2
Methylene blue	Much lower than true SaO_2
Fetal hemoglobin	No significant effect
Jaundice	No significant effect
Skin pigmentation	Variable[b]
Decreased perfusion	Variable[c]
Vasoconstriction	Variable[c]
Cardiac arrhythmias	Variable[c]
Hypothermia, shivering	Variable[c]

[a]See text for discussion.
[b]Studies report a variable effect, depending on the oximeter model and degree of skin pigmentation
[c]SpO_2 may stick on a falsely high or low reading

methemoglobin. This difference in technology means that a value of oxygen saturation at any point *can vary depending on how it is measured.* (If and when future generations of pulse oximeters have four-wavelength capability, the distinctions discussed herein will vanish.)

Clinical use of pulse oximetry

Pulse oximetry has been heralded as "arguably the most significant technological advance ever made in the monitoring of the well-being and safety of patients during anesthesia, recovery and critical care" (Severinghaus 1986) and as "the greatest advance in patient monitoring since electrocardiography" (Hanning & Alexander-Williams 1995). Clearly, this is a device with which all caregivers should be familiar. Much has been written about pulse oximetry, and reviews of the subject appear frequently (Council on Scientific Affairs 1993; Severinghaus & Kelleher 1992; Wahr & Tremper 1995).

Despite its acknowledged importance and simplicity of use, the pulse oximeter is often misused and its measurement misunderstood. The following points bear emphasis for anyone using a pulse oximeter (see also Table 6.3).

1. *Pulse oximetry does not differentiate carboxyhemoglobin from oxyhemoglobin* (Barker & Tremper 1987; Raemer et al. 1989; Hampson 1998). Pulse oximetry emits two wavelengths of light: 660 and 940 nm. Oxygenated hemoglobin (HbO_2) and deoxygenated hemoglobin (Hb) reflect these two wavelengths differently, allowing the oximeter to distinguish between them. Light transmission at 660 nm is mainly from HbO_2, and that at 940 nm is mainly from Hb. It turns out that COHb reflects just as much 660 nm wavelength light as HbO_2, and thus COHb is read as HbO_2 by the pulse oximeter. Thus, for example, a patient with a true SaO_2 of 85% plus 10% COHb will have a pulse oximetry SpO_2 reading of about 95%. For this reason, pulse oximeters should never be used to assess oxygenation in anyone who might have CO poisoning.
2. *Pulse oximetry does not reliably distinguish between oxygen desaturation from a low PaO_2 and from excess methemoglobin (MetHb).* Unlike carbon monoxide, MetHb does depress the SpO_2 reading, but not linearly (Baker et al. 1989; Eisenkraft 1988; Ralston et al. 1991; Watcha et al. 1989). MetHb decreases SpO_2, but the fall in SpO_2 is only by about one-half of the MetHb concentration, until a reading of 85% is reached; at this point, further increases in %MetHb do not lower the SpO_2 any further. Thus a pulse oximetry reading of 90% could represent
   a. A low PaO_2 causing oxygen desaturation of 10% (i.e., a true SaO_2 of 90%)
   b. Normal PaO_2 with methemoglobin in excess of 10%
   c. Some combination of a low PaO_2 and excess MetHb

As with CO, pulse oximeters should never be used to assess oxygenation in anyone who might have excess methemoglobin. Methylene blue is used to treat severe cases of excess methemoglobin; like many intravenous pigments, methylene blue causes a major drop in SpO_2 and is another reason to avoid the pulse oximeter altogether when managing this problem (Wahr & Tremper 1995).

3. *Clinically acceptable precision for SpO_2 is within ± 3% of the SaO_2, but the degree of precision varies among oximeter models* (Leasa 1992). Numerous studies have appeared correlating the precision or accuracy of different oximeters, and the results are variable. Knowing whether a particular model at a particular time is overestimating or underestimating oxygen saturation would require measuring SaO_2 (in a co-oximeter) at the time SpO_2 is also measured. This is obviously not practical or desirable. Instead, it seems prudent to assume that SpO_2 is overestimating SaO_2 and to take some action whenever SpO_2 falls below 93%. Such action would depend on the clinical situation, of course (e.g., close monitoring of vital signs and cardiac rhythm, adding or increasing supplemental O_2, beginning another treatment, checking an arterial blood gas).
4. *Pulse oximetry may give a false sense of security if the patient has adequate oxygen saturation but a declining PaO_2.* Because of the relatively flat portion of the O_2 dissociation curve above a PaO_2 of 60 mm Hg, and especially above 100 mm Hg, PaO_2 could drop significantly without an appreciable change in SpO_2 (Fig. 6.5).
5. *Pulse oximetry may give a false sense of security if the patient has adequate oxygen saturation but a rising $PaCO_2$.* A sedated or anesthetized patient receiving supplemental oxygen can maintain adequate SaO_2 *without adequate ventilation.* In the most extreme cases this is called *apneic oxygenation:* Diffusion of a high FIO_2 into the lungs maintains oxygenation, while the $PaCO_2$ rises to life-threatening levels (Ayas et al. 1998; Davidson & Hosie 1993; Hutton & Clutton-Brock 1993). Even with extreme acidosis, SaO_2 may stay in the normal range, especially if PaO_2 is maintained above normal (Fig. 6.6). (Oxygenation by diffusion is also used in the apnea test for brain death. Patients without spontaneous breathing, in whom neurologic exam points to brain death, are oxygenated by diffusion through an endotracheal tube without any mechanical breathing. Total absence of respirations when $PaCO_2$ reaches 60 mm Hg or higher, without confounding factors such as hypothermia or drug overdose, confirms brain death.)
6. *Pulse oximetry may be unreliable if there is poor tissue perfusion, vasoconstriction, or hypothermia.* This problem is most often seen in patients with decreased vas-

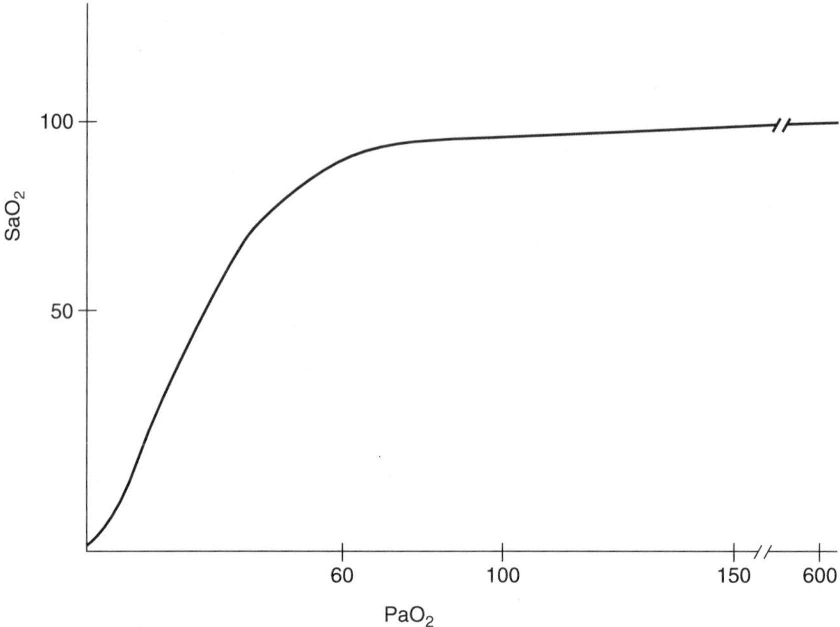

Figure 6.5. The oxygen dissociation curve is relatively flat above a PaO_2 of 60 mm Hg and is almost horizontal above a PaO_2 of 100 mm Hg. Thus a fall in PaO_2 that could be significant (in terms of gas exchange for the patient) can occur without an appreciable fall in SaO_2.

cular flow to the extremities. The machines work only if there is a strong pulse. With a weak pulse, the SpO_2 reading may stick on a falsely low or high value.

7. *There are limited studies on a host of other conditions that might interfere with pulse oximetry readings;* when in doubt, a blood gas with co-oximetry measurements should be obtained.

Nail polish. In some circumstances, dark nail polish can affect SpO_2, particularly dark black or blue colors. When this occurs, the polish appears to cause SpO_2 to be falsely low (Coté et al. 1988). In doubtful cases, one should simply remove the polish before taking a measurement.

Dark skin. Dark skin pigmentation may affect the SpO_2 value slightly with some oximeter models, but the results are inconsistent and no definitive variation has been published (Ralston et al. 1991; Ries et al. 1989; Zeballos & Weisman 1991).

Jaundice. Hyperbilirubinemia does not appear to affect pulse oximetry SpO_2 readings (Veyckemans et al. 1989).

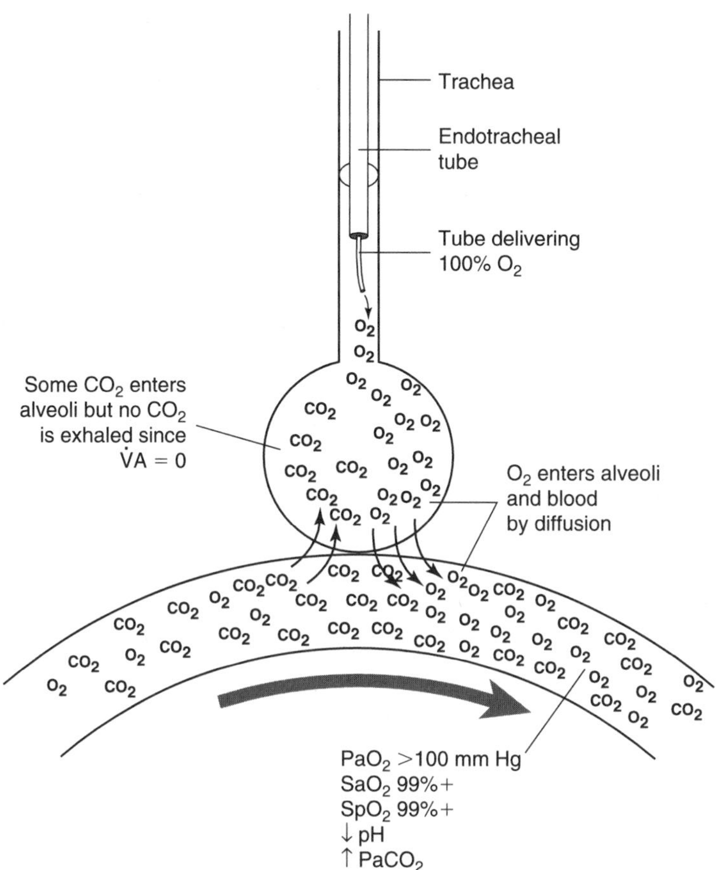

Figure 6.6. Apneic oxygenation. Diffusion of oxygen into the lungs through an endotracheal tube can oxygenate the blood even when there is zero alveolar ventilation. The PaO_2 may be normal or supernormal; as a result, SaO_2 and SpO_2 will stay in the normal range. If no other parameter of gas exchange is monitored, hypercapnia and progressive respiratory acidosis (↓pH, ↑$PaCO_2$) will be missed. Note that although some CO_2 diffuses into the alveolar spaces, there is no exchange of CO_2 with the atmosphere because there is no alveolar ventilation.

Fetal hemoglobin does not appear to affect SpO_2 readings. Paradoxically, however, it can interfere with co-oximetry readings (Barker & Tremper 1987; Lindberg et al. 1995).

8. *Pulse oximetry can be misused by people unfamiliar with how it works and what it measures.* A 1994 study showed that doctors and nurses were surprisingly ignorant about some basic oximetry principles and made serious errors in interpretation of readings (Stoneham et al. 1994). For example,

30% of doctors and 93% of nurses thought the oximeter measured PaO_2 or oxygen content. In the same study, only one doctor and one nurse (3% of each sample) knew that an oximeter requires pulsatile flow of blood under the sensor.

Of course, the pulse oximeter is so simple to use that anyone can record an SpO_2, whereas only trained laboratory personnel can run a blood sample through a co-oximeter. This ease of use invites misapplication. I have seen health care personnel at all levels—physicians, nurses, therapists—unintentionally chart a false reading because they were unfamiliar with the device and the pitfalls mentioned above. This problem is compounded when a charted value is taken as reliable by other health care workers, when in fact it may be totally erroneous.

Pulse oximetry—examples in practice

Pulse oximetry is most useful for following SpO_2 over time (continuous reading), particularly when the SpO_2 has been correlated with at least one direct measurement of SaO_2. In this setting, pulse oximetry can often obviate the need for frequent blood gas monitoring. Conversely, pulse oximetry may alert one to the need for blood gas measurement; for example, when the SpO_2 reading is lower than expected in a patient receiving supplemental O_2.

A patient in the ER has a blood gas drawn at the same time as a pulse oximetry measurement. The arterial PaO_2 is 77 mm Hg (breathing room air). Below are three values for arterial oxygen saturation, with information about how each was determined.

95% calculated from PaO2 value
98% from pulse oximeter
85% from co-oximeter

Why do these values disagree and which is the most reliable?

This question illustrates the three ways oxygen saturation is usually obtained. By far the most reliable method is direct measurement of an arterial sample in the co-oximeter. Using four wavelengths of light, the co-oximeter makes direct measurements of oxyhemoglobin, carboxyhemoglobin, and methemoglobin and so gives the only true measurement of SaO_2. Pulse oximetry, on the other hand, includes carboxyhemoglobin and a variable amount of any excess methemoglobin in its reading of oxygen saturation and so will *overestimate* SaO_2 in the presence of excess dyshemoglobins.

As for the calculated SaO_2, it is only reliable if nothing else but oxygen is binding to hemoglobin, which you can't know from just the PaO_2. In this example, the patient actually had 10% carboxyhemoglobin and 2% methemoglobin, so the calculated SaO_2 of 95% was misleading. In summary, it is always important to know where your oxygen saturation value is coming from and to interpret it accordingly.

A 55-year-old man is hospitalized following a heart attack. The arterial blood gas while breathing room air shows a PaO_2 of 84 mm Hg and a measured SaO_2 of 95%; the initial SpO_2 is 96%. He is started on nasal oxygen and cardiac medications and is monitored for cardiac rhythm and pulse oximetry. Two days later, his SpO_2 is 88%. He is in no distress, his lungs are clear on exam, and the chest x-ray is normal. The nurse thinks he has a bluish tinge to his skin that was not present on admission. How would you explain the change from an SpO_2 of 96 to 88% over the two days?

The pulse oximeter SpO_2 could be low because of a low PaO_2, but there was no reason to suspect this; his pulmonary status had not changed, and he was receiving supplemental oxygen. His medications, however, included a long-acting nitrate for coronary artery disease. The low SpO_2 necessitated measurement of arterial blood gases. PaO_2 was increased at 123 mm Hg (on nasal oxygen); but a low SaO_2 was confirmed (87%), and methemoglobin was measured at 12.2%. The excess MetHb was attributed to a side effect of the nitrate medication, and his skin was bluish because of this dyshemoglobin. Without excess MetHb, his SaO_2 would have been about 96%. The nitrate was discontinued, and two days later his pulse oximetry SpO_2 was 98%, while a co-oximeter-measured SaO_2 was 95% and MetHb 2.4%.

Clinical Problem 6.4. A patient comes to the emergency department without assistance, complaining of dyspnea and headaches. Pulse oximetry shows an SpO_2 of 94%. How much excess CO could be in this patient's blood?

Clinical Problem 6.5. A patient comatose from CO poisoning is brought to the hospital. Initial arterial blood gas on room air reveals pH = 7.30, $PaCO_2$ = 30 mm Hg, PaO_2 = 85 mm Hg, SaO_2 = 45%, COHb = 52%, and hemoglobin content = 15 g/dL. Calculate the patient's arterial PO_2 and oxygen content under each of the conditions listed below. In each situation, assume no change in $PaCO_2$, $P(A\text{–}a)O_2$ = 50 mm Hg, and barometric pressure = 760 mm Hg.

a. 80% oxygen by face mask; CO level down to 45%
b. Intubated, on 100% FIO_2; CO level down to 40%
c. In a hyperbaric chamber at 2 atm pressure (= 1520 mm Hg), on 100% FIO_2; CO level down to 40%
d. In a hyperbaric chamber at 3 atm pressure (=2280 mm Hg), FIO_2 100%; CO level down to 30%.

Clinical Problem 6.6. With 100% inspired oxygen, approximately how many atmospheres of pressure are necessary to provide an arterial oxygen content in the plasma phase that would equal the total arterial content available when breathing room air at sea level? Calculate your answer for a patient with normal lungs and hemoglobin content; assume a $P(A\text{–}a)O_2$ of 50 mm Hg.

a. 4
b. 6
c. 9
d. 15
e. 20

Clinical Problem 6.7. A patient with no history of respiratory disease has endoscopy for a stomach problem. He is given 3 L/min nasal O_2, and SpO_2 is monitored with pulse oximetry. At the beginning of the procedure, SpO_2 is 99%; halfway through the endoscopy SpO_2 is down to 91%. The patient shows no respiratory distress. What is your explanation for the change in SpO_2? What should be done?

ANSWERS TO CLINICAL PROBLEMS

6.1. For these comparisons you needed to check Figure 6.2 for the SaO_2 values for the given pH and PaO_2. (Expect some slight variation in the SaO_2 values from those listed below.) The amount of oxygen contributed by the dissolved fraction is negligible and will not affect the answer.

a.

Patient 1: $CaO_2 = 0.93 \times 10 \times 1.34 = 12.5$ mL O_2/dL
Patient 2: $CaO_2 = 0.89 \times 10 \times 1.34 = 11.9$ mL O_2/dL

Patient 2 is slightly more hypoxemic.

b.

Patient 1: $CaO_2 = 0.92 \times 15 \times 1.34 = 18.5$ mL O_2/dL
Patient 2: $CaO_2 = 0.92 \times 15 \times 1.34 = 18.5$ mL O_2/dL

The patients have equal amounts of hemoglobin-bound oxygen content.

c.

Patient 1: $CaO_2 = 0.90 \times 12 \times 1.34 = 14.5$ mL O_2/dL
Patient 2: $CaO_2 = 0.80 \times 12 \times 1.34 = 12.9$ mL O_2/dL

Patient 2 is more hypoxemic.

d.

Patient 1: $CaO_2 = 0.98 \times 12 \times 1.34 = 15.8$ mL O_2/dL
Patient 2: $CaO_2 = 0.90 \times 12 \times 1.34 = 14.5$ mL O_2/dL

Patient 2 is more hypoxemic.

6.2.

pH	PCO_2	P_{50}
7.26	60	31
7.32	50	29.5
7.40	40	27
7.48	30	24.5
7.56	20	22

6.3. For this problem you have to find the SaO_2 for some of the PaO_2 values from a standard oxygen dissociation curve, then subtract the CO level to arrive at the true SaO_2.

a.

Patient 1: $CaO_2 = 0.78 \times 15 \times 1.34 = 15.7$ mL O_2/dL
Patient 2: $CaO_2 = 0.98 \times 12 \times 1.34 = 15.8$ mL O_2/dL

The oxygen contents are almost identical; therefore, neither patient is more *hypoxemic*. Patient 1, however, with 20% CO, is more *hypoxic* than patient 2 because of the left shift of the O_2 dissociation curve caused by the excess CO.

b.

Patient 1: $CaO_2 = 0.87 \times 15 \times 1.34 = 17.5$ mL O_2/dL
Patient 2: $CaO_2 = 0.85 \times 15 \times 1.34 = 17.1$ mL O_2/dL

A PaO_2 of 90 mm Hg with pH of 7.20 gives an SaO_2 of approximately 92%; subtracting 5% COHb from this value gives a true SaO_2 of 87%, used in the CaO_2 calculation of patient 1. A PaO_2 of 50 mm Hg with normal pH gives an SaO_2 of 85%. Thus patient 2 is slightly more hypoxemic.

c.

Patient 1: $CaO_2 = 0.90 \times 5 \times 1.34 = 6.0$ mL O_2/dL
Patient 2: $CaO_2 = 0.78 \times 15 \times 1.34 = 15.7$ mL O_2/dL

Patient 1 is more hypoxemic, because of severe anemia.

d.

Patient 1: $CaO_2 = 0.87 \times 10 \times 1.34 = 11.7$ mL O_2/dL
Patient 2: $CaO_2 = 0.83 \times 15 \times 1.34 = 16.7$ mL O_2/dL

Patient 1 is more hypoxemic.

6.4. Virtually any amount of CO could be in this patient's blood (although the fact that he came to the ER without assistance suggests the level is $< 40\%$). Pulse oximetry reads carboxyhemoglobin and oxyhemoglobin together and reports the two values as SpO_2.

6.5. Answers for this problem require the use of both the alveolar gas and the oxygen content equations. Because of the high FIO_2 values, the factor 1.2 is dropped from the alveolar gas equation (Chapter 4). Also, we can assume that $SaO_2 = 100\%$ minus the %COHb. Unlike the other problems presented so far, here we cannot ignore the contribution of dissolved oxygen to the total oxygen content.

a.

$PAO_2 = 0.8(713) - 30$ mm Hg $= 540$ mm Hg
$PaO_2 = 540 - 50 = 490$ mm Hg
$CaO_2 = (15 \times 0.55 \times 1.34) + (0.003 \times 490) = 11.1 + 1.5 = 12.6$ mL O_2/dL

b.

$PAO_2 = 1.0(760 - 47) - 30$ mm Hg $= 683$ mm Hg

$PaO_2 = 683 - 50 = 633$ mm Hg
$CaO_2 = (15 \times 0.60 \times 1.34) + (0.003 \times 633) = 12.1 + 1.9 = 14.0$ mL O_2/dL

c.

$PAO_2 = 1.0(1520 - 47) - 30$ mm Hg $= 1443$ mm Hg
$PaO_2 = 1443 - 50 = 1393$ mm Hg
$CaO_2 = (15 \times 0.60 \times 1.34) + (0.003 \times 1393) = 12.1 + 4.2 = 16.3$ mL O_2/dL

d.

$PAO_2 = 1.0(2280 - 47) - 30$ mm Hg $= 2203$ mm Hg
$PaO_2 = 2203 - 50 = 2153$ mm Hg
$CaO_2 = (15 \times 0.70 \times 1.34) + (0.003 \times 2153) = 14.1 + 6.5 = 20.6$ mL O_2/dL

6.6. c. Assuming normal ventilation ($PaCO_2 = 40$ mm Hg) and a $P(A–a)O_2$ of 50 mm Hg, the following calculations show that 1 atm of pressure places about 1.9 mL O_2/dL dissolved oxygen in the blood when breathing 100% oxygen.

$$PAO_2 = 1.0(760 - 47) - 40 \text{ mm Hg} = 673 \text{ mm Hg}$$
$$PaO_2 = PAO_2 - 50 \text{ mm Hg} = 623 \text{ mm Hg}$$
$$\text{Dissolved } O_2 \text{ content} = 0.003 - 623 = 1.87 \text{ mL } O_2/\text{dL}$$

Each additional atmosphere delivers a slightly higher O_2 content because the $PaCO_2$ and water vapor pressure are subtracted only once. Thus the next atmosphere of oxygen pressure can contribute

$$0.003 \times 760 \text{ mm Hg} = 2.3 \text{ mL } O_2/\text{dL}$$

Normal blood oxygen content is about 20 mL O_2/dL. Because each atmosphere at 100% FIO_2 delivers slightly over 2 mL O_2/dL to the blood, the correct answer is 9 atm. To check this answer, assume someone is breathing 100% oxygen at 9 atm (strictly hypothetical; this would be extremely toxic and quickly fatal). Then:

$$9 \text{ atm} \times 760 \text{ mm Hg/atm} = 6840 \text{ mm Hg}$$
$$PAO_2 = 1.00\ (6840 - 47) - 40 = 6753 \text{ mm Hg}$$
$$O_2 \text{ content (plasma phase only)} = 0.003 \times 6753 = 20.26 \text{ mL } O_2/\text{dL}$$

6.7. When someone with a normal respiratory system breathes supplemental oxygen, the SpO_2 should be close to 100%. A fall in SpO_2 from 99 to 91% could be the result of a precipitous fall in PaO_2 (e.g., from pulmonary aspiration), but such a condition would likely be accompanied by some respiratory distress. A more likely explanation is development of methemoglobinemia from topical airway anesthetic; such anesthetics are commonly used to facilitate insertion of the endoscope. The methemoglobin imparts a dark color to the blood, which shows up clinically as a bluish tinge to the skin; this is not cyanosis from deoxygenated hemoglobin (which must be at least 5 g/dL to be manifest) but is instead directly owing to the color of methemoglobin.

Once methemoglobinemia is suspected, the endoscopy procedure should be aborted, and the patient examined for a change in skin color, a bluish tinge is always present with any significant increase in methemoglobinemia. At the same time, the FIO_2 should be increased (by switching to a high-flow oxygen face mask), and the patient monitored carefully over the next 24 h, both clinically and with arterial blood gas measurements (*not* with pulse oximetry). Specific treatment with a reducing agent (e.g., methylene blue) is not necessary unless the methemoglobin continues to increase and poses a threat to the patient. There is no minimal threshold that demands treatment, but it should be strongly considered if the methemoglobin exceeds 15%.

CHAPTER

7

pH, $PaCO_2$, Electrolytes, and Acid–Base Status

THE HENDERSON–HASSELBALCH EQUATION AND pH

Among the three physiologic processes assessed by blood gas data, acid–base is perhaps the most complicated. Oxygenation and ventilation problems can often be assessed by a single abnormal variable (e.g., PaO_2 or $PaCO_2$) and almost always arise from impairment of a single organ system (respiratory). By contrast, acid–base disorders require knowledge of two or more variables, and they may arise from renal, pulmonary, and/or gastrointestinal impairment or from exogenous chemicals and poisons.

Carbon dioxide, a byproduct of metabolism, combines with water in the blood to form carbonic acid, H_2CO_3. Carbonic acid quickly dissociates into hydrogen ions and bicarbonate. These reactions are reversible, i.e., they may go either way.

$$CO_2 + H_2O \leftrightarrow H_2CO_3 \leftrightarrow H^+ + HCO_3^-$$

The concentration of hydrogen ions is related to the concentration of carbonic acid and bicarbonate. The Henderson–Hasselbalch (H–H) equation defines the hydrogen ion concentration in terms of pH as follows:

$$pH = pK + \log \frac{[HCO_3^-]}{[H_2CO_3]}$$

where

pK = negative logarithm of the dissociation constant for carbonic acid (6.1)
pH = negative logarithm of hydrogen ion concentration ($[H^+]$) in nanomoles/liter (nMol/L)

Almost all H_2CO_3 in the blood is in the form of dissolved CO_2. To obtain a quantity for the denominator of the equation, $PaCO_2$ is multiplied by its solubility coefficient, 0.03 mEq/L/mm Hg. Thus we obtain the more familiar form of the H–H equation.

$$pH = pK + \log \frac{HCO_3^-}{0.03(PaCO_2)}$$

Using units that express concentration, what is the normal HCO_3^-:$PaCO_2$ ratio in the H–H equation?

a. 2.4:4.0
b. 1:2
c. 2:1
d. 10:1
e. 20:1

Normal HCO_3^- is 24 mEq/L and normal $PaCO_2$ is 40 mm Hg; this $PaCO_2$ value times 0.03 = 1.2 mEq/L, so the normal ratio is 20:1. The logarithm of 20 is 1.3 which, when added to the pK value of 6.1, gives the normal pH of 7.4.

Many people view pH, which is unitless, as an unnecessarily confusing term; not only does pH correlate *inversely* with [H^+] but small numerical changes reflect large changes in [H^+] (Table 7.1). In years past, there was much debate on whether pH should be discarded in favor of [H^+] as the clinical term for acidity (Campbell & Rip 1962; Hills 1973; Lennon & Lemann

TABLE 7.1. pH AND HYDROGEN ION CONCENTRATION

BLOOD pH	[H^+] (nMol/L)	CHANGE FROM NORMAL (%)
Acidemia		
7.00	100	+150
7.10	80	+100
7.30	50	+25
Normal		
7.40	40	
Alkalemia		
7.52	30	−25
7.70	20	−50
8.00	10	−75

1966). Whatever the merits of this argument, pH has remained in worldwide use and seems in no danger of yielding to $[H^+]$ in blood gas reports.

Table 7.1 shows the corresponding $[H^+]$ values for pH from 7.00 to 8.00 and the percent change between selected values. A pH of 7.40 = 40 nM/L $[H^+]$. An 0.1 unit *decrease* in pH from 7.40 to 7.30 represents a 25% *increase* in $[H^+]$. A similar percentage change in serum sodium would raise its value from a normal 140 to 175 mEq/L!

Although practically everyone entering the clinical arena is taught the H–H equation at some point, outside blood gas labs the equation is seldom (if ever) used to calculate pH or any other variable. Why then such emphasis on this admittedly complicated equation? Clinical importance of the H–H equation relates to the following:

- The bicarbonate system is quantitatively the largest buffering system in the extracellular fluid; its buffer components (HCO_3^- and $PaCO_2$) instantly reflect any blood acid–base disturbance.
- The three variables in the H–H equation are easily measured (or two can be measured and the third calculated).
- The simple proportion in the equation

$$pH \approx \frac{HCO_3^-}{PaCO_2}$$

can be used to describe the four primary acid–base disorders. The *change*, in both degree and direction, of the two buffer components is the key to understanding acid–base disorders.

What is the pH of a blood sample with HCO_3^- = 36 mEq/L and $PaCO_2$ = 60 mm Hg?

a. 7.1
b. 7.3
c. 7.4
d. 7.5
e. Indeterminate without more data

I wrote earlier that a calculator was not required when reading this book, so don't bother looking for one to calculate the logarithm in the H–H equation. In this question, both HCO_3^- and $PaCO_2$ are increased 50% above normal, but since the ratio of the two values is unchanged, the logarithm of the ratio and resulting pH are also unchanged. The correct answer is, therefore, 7.4.

What is the pH of a blood sample with $HCO_3^- = 16$ mEq/L?

a. 7.1
b. 7.3
c. 7.4
d. 7.4
e. Indeterminate without more data

The answer is indeterminate. You need to know two of the three H–H variables to obtain the third. In this example, the blood could be acidemic or alkalemic.

What is the pH of a blood sample with $HCO_3^- = 24$ mEq/L and $PaCO_2 =$ 80 mm Hg?

a. 7.1
b. 7.3
c. 7.4
d. 7.4
e. 7.6

You could calculate pH from the H–H equation but it is unnecessary. A normal HCO_3^- with twice the normal $PaCO_2$ will make the blood very acidic, far more than just pH 7.3, which is only 25% above baseline acidity (Table 7.1). The only reasonable answer among the choices given is pH 7.1.

VENOUS CO_2—WHAT IT MEASURES AND HOW TO USE IT

In the blood gas lab, $PaCO_2$ and pH are measured and HCO_3^- is calculated from the Henderson–Hasselbalch equation. By contrast, chemistry labs *measure* bicarbonate in venous blood as a component of the serum electrolytes. What they measure, however, is often labeled not bicarbonate but "CO_2." Thus the four routinely measured electrolytes in venous blood are Na^+, K^+, Cl^-, and CO_2 (Fig. 7.1).

A

	COLLECTION DATE		08MAY98
	TIME DRAWN		0904
RESULT	REF RANGE	UNITS	
FIO2		%	35
LITER FLOW		L/M	
MODE			VENT
TYPE			ART
- - - -Blood Gas- - -			
PH	[7.35–7.45]		7.43
PCO2	[35–45]	MM HG	35
PO2	[60–100]	MM HG	**143 H**
HCO3−	[22–26]	MEQ/L	23
SAO2 MEAS	[93–100]	%	97
SAO2 CALC	[93–100]	%	
HB	[12.0–16.0]	G/DL	**8.7 L**
COHB	[0.0–3.0]	%	1.5
METHB	[0.0–2.0]	%	1.2
O2 CONT	[16–22]	VOL %	**12 L**
BASE EXC	[−2.0–2.0]	MEQ/L	−0.1

B 08MAY98

	SODIUM	POTASSIUM	CHLORIDE	CO2
REF RANGE	[135–145]	[3.5–5.0]	[98–107]	[24–30]
UNITS	MEQ/L	MEQ/L	MEQ/L	MEQ/L
0715	145	4.2	102	**22 L**

Figure 7.1. Actual arterial blood gas results (**A**) and venous (serum) electrolytes (**B**) for a patient who was receiving mechanical ventilation (VENT) with an FIO_2 of 35%. Note that in the blood gas report, bicarbonate is calculated from the pH and $PaCO_2$ using the Henderson–Hasselbalch equation and the normal range is 22–26 mEq/L. For electrolytes, venous CO_2 is a direct measurement and normal range is 24–30 mEq/L. The venous CO_2 incorporates both venous bicarbonate and dissolved CO_2. The lab's computer flags abnormally low or high values and prints them in boldface.

The venous or serum CO_2 includes both the true bicarbonate (the numerator in the H–H equation) *and* the mEq/L of CO_2 contributed by dissolved CO_2 (which is the determinant of PCO_2). When dissolved CO_2 exerts a normal *partial pressure* of 46 mm Hg in venous blood, its *quantity* in the blood is

$$0.03 \text{ mEq/L/mm Hg} \times 46 \text{ mm Hg} = 1.38 \text{ mEq/L}$$

Furthermore, venous bicarbonate is slightly higher than the arterial bicarbonate (by 1–3 mEq/L). Thus what the chemistry lab routinely measures as

CO_2 in venous blood is different quantitatively, by approximately 2–4 mEq/L, from what the blood gas lab calculates in arterial blood as HCO_3^-.

The clinical chemistry lab measures, in the serum fraction of venous blood, *both* the actual bicarbonate (the numerator in the H–H equation) and the quantity of dissolved CO_2 (the denominator in the H–H equation) and reports the result as CO_2 (or sometimes "total CO_2") in mEq/L. As can be seen in Figure 7.1, the normal venous CO_2 ranges from 24 to 30 mEq/L, whereas the calculated arterial HCO_3^- ranges from 22 to 26 mEq/L. (The venous value obviously should not be confused with $PaCO_2$, which is the partial pressure of *arterial* CO_2 as measured in the blood gas lab.)

Although the measured venous CO_2 should be within 2–4 mEq/L of the calculated arterial HCO_3^-, the difference is often greater and can occur *in both directions*. Table 7.2 lists some reasons why the two values differ (and sometimes significantly) and why either value may be higher or lower than the other.

Clinical Problem 7.1. A 54-year-old man is hospitalized with congestive heart failure. The blood gas lab reports arterial pH = 7.52, $PaCO_2$ = 44 mm Hg, and HCO_3^- = 34 mEq/L. A venous CO_2 measured at the same time is 24 mEq/L. How would you assess his acid–base status?

TABLE 7.2. REASONS WHY THE CALCULATED ARTERIAL HCO_3^- MAY DIFFER FROM THE MEASURED VENOUS CO_2

1. Venous HCO_3^- normally runs slightly higher than arterial HCO_3^-
2. Arterial HCO_3^- is calculated using a pK value of 6.1; venous value is measured as part of the total CO_2 (which includes contribution of PCO_2)
3. The true pK may vary from the assumed value of 6.1 in critically ill patients (Hood 1982)
4. Arterial and venous blood are usually drawn at different times, and the patient's acid–base state may have changed in interim.
5. Venous blood may sit in a test tube open to the air before it is measured, thereby losing some CO_2 to diffusion.
6. The blood-drawing technique may alter venous CO_2, e.g., tourniquet placement may create a transient lactic acidosis, lowering the venous HCO_3^-
7. If pH and/or $PaCO_2$ are inaccurately measured, the calculated HCO_3^- will be inaccurate as well

Although two of the three H–H variables are needed to determine the third, an isolated value can be clinically useful. If any one of the three H–H variables is truly abnormal, the patient must have an acid–base disturbance of some type. Therefore, assuming no lab or transcription error, **a high or low calculated HCO_3^-** or measured serum CO_2 indicates an acid–base disorder. The possibilities are as follows:

Diagnostic possibilities for high and low bicarbonate/serum CO_2

Elevated HCO_3^- or serum CO_2

a. Metabolic alkalosis and/or
b. Bicarbonate retention as compensation for respiratory acidosis

Reduced HCO_3^- or serum CO_2

a. Metabolic acidosis and/or
b. Bicarbonate excretion as compensation for respiratory alkalosis

Since serum electrolytes in venous blood are measured far more often than arterial blood gases, serum CO_2 is often the first clue to an underlying acid–base disorder. Overlooking an abnormal CO_2 value can lead to serious clinical error. In Chapter 3, I presented the case of an elderly patient given a sedative when the physician mistakenly assumed she was hyperventilating. At the time the sedative was ordered, there were two venous CO_2 measurements in her hospital chart, both 34 mEq/L, but no arterial blood gas values.

From the limited information provided, what do you think explains that patient's elevated venous CO_2?

a. Metabolic alkalosis
b. Respiratory acidosis with renal compensation
c. Normal for an elderly patient
d. Laboratory error

Abnormality of a single H–H variable can arise from *two or more* acid–base disorders. For example, the increased HCO_3^- or serum CO_2 as in this patient can occur from metabolic alkalosis or respiratory acidosis, or both. A lab error, always a possibility, is less likely when two separate measurements are in close agreement. No blood gases had been measured before the sedative was ordered; perhaps it was assumed that her elevated serum CO_2 reflected only a mild metabolic alkalosis, from prior diuretic therapy. She also had a long smoking history, so respiratory acidosis was another possible explanation for the elevated CO_2. In fact, her CO_2 did reflect chronic respiratory acidosis with renal compensation.

When she arrived at the intensive care unit, her pH was 7.07, $PaCO_2$ was 83 mm Hg, and calculated HCO_3^- was 23 mEq/L, values that reflected a worsening of previously unrecognized respiratory acidosis *plus* a new metabolic acidosis (lactic acid was elevated because of poor organ perfusion). Her distress just before the ICU transfer was related to increasing respiratory acidosis and dyspnea.

Finally, note that, although there are two possibilities each for high or low serum CO_2, as a practical matter a very high or very low value indicates a metabolic disorder. Compensation for respiratory alkalosis seldom lowers CO_2 below 12 mEq/L, and compensation for respiratory acidosis seldom raises CO_2 above 45 mEq/L. Thus if you find a serum CO_2 below 12 mEq/L there almost assuredly is a metabolic acidosis; similarly, a serum CO_2 above 45 mEq/L almost assuredly indicates a metabolic alkalosis.

ELECTROLYTES AND THE ANION GAP

Although the focus of this book is on arterial blood gases, a discussion of routine serum electrolytes is also important, for they are vital to blood gas interpretation in many situations. The above discussion on venous CO_2 highlights one interrelationship between electrolytes and blood gases.

An electrolyte abnormality is often the *first* laboratory sign of an acid–base disorder. As a minimum, electrolytes used to calculate the anion gap—sodium, chloride, and bicarbonate (measured as serum CO_2)—should always be measured in any patient with a blood gas or acid–base abnormality. Since potassium is often deranged in acid–base disorders, it should also be examined.

The anion gap (AG) calculation is the sum of routinely measured cations minus routinely measured anions:

$$(Na^+ + K^+) - (Cl^- + HCO_3^-)$$

However, because K^+ is a small value numerically, it is usually omitted from the AG equation; so that, as most commonly used, it takes the following form:

$$AG = Na^+ - (Cl^- + HCO_3^-)$$

Although this is the equation most often published in articles and textbooks, for reasons discussed above, the equation incorporates not the calculated arterial HCO_3^- but the measured venous CO_2. To add to the confusion, some labs report the measured venous value as HCO_3^- and other labs as CO_2. Whatever the label for the reported venous value, *that* is the one you should use in calculating AG, because normal values are based on the venous electrolyte measurements. Throughout this book, the anion gap will be calculated as

$$AG = Na^+ - (Cl^- + CO_2)$$

The normal AG calculated in this manner (without K^+) is 12 ± 4 mEq/L. The anion gap exists simply because not *all* electrolytes are routinely measured. Normally, there is an electrochemical balance, so that the sum of all negatively charged electrolytes (anions) equals the sum of all positively charged electrolytes (cations); however, several anions are not routinely measured, leading to the anion gap. The anion gap is thus an artifact of measurement, and not a physiologic reality.

Table 7.3 lists all the cations and anions with their normal serum values. Note that if they were all measured, there would be no gap, because positives equal negatives. Because only Na^+, K^+, Cl^-, and CO_2 are routinely measured, however, there is an anion gap; the gap exists because more anions are left *unmeasured* than are cations (Oh & Carroll 1977). Finally, because K^+ is usually not used in the calculation, the normal anion gap is about 12 mEq/L.

One important technical aspect should be noted about anion gap measurement before discussing its clinical utility. There can be variation in the normal AG, depending on the technology used to measure electrolytes (Sadjadi 1995; Winter et al. 1990). Although the technical aspects of measurement are beyond the scope of this book, it is important to realize that some clinical labs use a method that gives a *lower* normal range (e.g., 3–11 mEq/L) (Winter et al. 1990). Always use the normal AG for your lab, and recognize that it may well vary from the 12 ± 4 mEq/L used in this book. As with any lab test, if you understand what is being measured, then even without knowing the technical aspects of the measurement you can use the information effectively.

The anion gap can be normal, low, or high; and each result has a different clinical implication.

- *Normal anion gap.* In this case there is no lab evidence for anion gap acidosis. This result does not always rule out an anion gap acidosis but certainly makes that diagnosis unlikely.
- *Very low or negative anion gap.* There are several reasons why this can occur, including:

TABLE 7.3. ANIONS AND CATIONS IN SERUM.

Because of the electrochemical balance, the concentrations of serum cations and anions are the same. In the routine measurement of electrolytes, however, more anions are unmeasured than are cations; this leads to an expected anion gap. As typically calculated, the anion gap is based on only three electrolytes: sodium, chloride, and bicarbonate (or serum CO_2).

ANIONS		CATIONS	
ELECTROLYTE	VALUE (MEQ/L)	ELECTROLYTE	VALUE (MEQ/L)
	All anions and cations		
Proteins	15	Calcium	5
Organic acids	5	Magnesium	1.5
Phosphates	2	Potassium	4.5
Sulfates	1	Sodium	140
Chloride	104		
Bicarbonate	24		
Totals	*151*		*151*
	Anions and cations used to calculate the anion gap		
Chloride + bicarbonate	128	Sodium	140
	Difference = 12		

Halide ion measured as chloride, as seen in bromism (some cough medications contain dextromethorphan bromide);

Excess unmeasured cation, as seen in lithium toxicity;

Reduction in the unmeasured anions, as seen in hypoproteinemia (a 1 g/dL decrease in serum albumin causes a 2.5 mEq/L drop in the AG); and

Presence of abnormal, positively charged proteins (paraproteins), as may be seen in multiple myeloma.

- Except for hypoproteinemia, conditions that cause a reduced or negative anion gap are relatively rare compared to those associated with an elevated anion gap.
- *Elevated anion gap.* The patient may have an anion gap metabolic acidosis (see Table 8.1); the higher the gap above normal, the more likely this will be the case.

All excess anions in the blood are buffered by bicarbonate, and this is why an elevated AG usually indicates a state of metabolic acidosis (Emmett & Narris 1977; Gabow et al. 1980; Gabow 1985; Narins & Emmett 1980; Oster et al. 1988). **This statement is true even if the actual measured venous CO_2 is normal or above normal.**

When AG is increased, one or more of the conditions listed in Table 8.1 should be considered. The most common causes are lactic acidosis, renal failure (build up of organic acids normally excreted by the kidney), and diabetic ketoacidosis. Less common causes include an overdose of acetylsalicylic acid (aspirin) and the breakdown products of some ingested poisons (ethylene glycol and methanol).

> **Clinical Problem 7.2.** A patient with a $PaCO_2$ of 50 mm Hg and an anion gap of 20 mEq/L has the following electrolyte values: $Na^+ = 145$ mEq/L and $Cl^- = 104$ mEq/L. From this information, how could you calculate the pH?

One problem with the anion gap is deciding what value is truly abnormal. In the majority of patients with an anion gap between 16 and 20 mEq/L, no specific anion gap acidosis can be diagnosed. Above 20 mEq/L, the probability of a true anion gap acidosis increases markedly (and is 100% if the AG is above 29 mEq/L). As a practical matter, you should consider an AG $\geq$ 20 mEq/L as reflecting an anion gap metabolic acidosis and search for the cause.

A 42-year-old man is admitted to the hospital with dehydration and hypotension. Electrolytes show $Na^+ = 165$ mEq/L, $K^+ = 4.0$ mEq/L, $CO_2 =$ 32 mEq/L, and $Cl^- = 112$ mEq/L. No arterial blood gas is obtained. Does this patient have metabolic acidosis?

Yes. His anion gap is $165 - (32 + 112) = 21$ mEq/L. Despite the fact that CO_2 is elevated (reflecting a metabolic *alkalosis* from dehydration), there is *also* a slight metabolic *acidosis*; the acidosis is from lactic acidosis, a result of the hypotension and poor organ perfusion. The coexistence of metabolic acidosis and metabolic alkalosis is discussed further in the following section and in Chapter 8.

More on examining electrolytes for mixed metabolic disorders: the bicarbonate gap

The subject of mixed acid–base disorders based on arterial blood gas interpretation is introduced in Chapter 8. However, mixed *metabolic* disorders alone can often be diagnosed from the serum electrolytes, as indicated in the previous example—an increased anion gap in the setting of an elevated venous CO_2.

In less obvious cases, the coexistence of two metabolic acid–base disorders may be apparent by calculating the *difference* between the change in anion gap and change in serum CO_2 (Haber 1991; Wrenn 1990). This calculation is called the *bicarbonate gap.*[*]

$$\text{Bicarbonate gap} = \Delta AG - \Delta CO_2$$

where

$$\Delta AG = \text{patient's AG} - 12 \text{ mEq/L}$$
$$\Delta CO_2 = 27 \text{ mEq/L} - \text{patient's } CO_2$$

If an anion gap acidosis is the only acid–base abnormality, there should be a 1:1 correlation between the rise in anion gap and the fall in bicarbonate (measured as serum CO_2); i.e., the normal difference between rise in AG and fall in serum CO_2 should be zero. For example, if AG goes up by 10 mEq/L (to 24 mEq/L) then serum CO_2 should go down by 10 mEq/L (to 17 mEq/L); in this case:

$$\Delta AG - \Delta CO_2 = 10 - 10 = 0 \text{ bicarbonate gap}$$

Elevated AG with a significant variation of bicarbonate gap from zero, either positive or negative, suggests that the patient has a mixed acid–base disorder: anion gap acidosis plus another disorder, such as metabolic alkalosis (+ bicarbonate gap) or hyperchloremic metabolic acidosis (− bicarbonate gap).

Although the concept is sound, one problem with the bicarbonate gap is deciding the outer limits of normal. Because we don't know a given patient's baseline AG and serum CO_2, deviations may be more or less significant than presumed. The problem is compounded by the fact that there is no accepted standard on how to calculate ΔAG and ΔCO_2. For example, some authors calculate ΔAG by subtracting the measured AG from the upper limit of the normal AG (e.g., 16 mEq/L), whereas others subtract it from the mean AG (e.g, 12 mEq/L).

For this reason, as well as the variations inherent in the underlying electrolyte values, there is no accepted normal value for the bicarbonate gap. Some

---

*Terms for the difference between the change in anion gap and change in serum CO_2 include *bicarbonate gap, delta gap,* and *deviation from the 1:1 correlation.* In this book I use *bicarbonate gap,* because that term seems closest to describing the basic concept.

authors call the bicarbonate gap abnormal if it deviates more than ± 6 mEq/L (Wrenn 1990), whereas others propose a deviation of more than ± 8 mEq/L as abnormal (Paulson & Gadallah 1993).

More important than a precise abnormal value is the concept of how the bicarbonate gap is used to diagnose mixed acid–base disorders. For didactic purposes, I will call abnormal any bicarbonate gap > 6 mEq/L or < −6 mEq/L, meaning it should prompt a close search for the cause. The more abnormal the bicarbonate gap value, the more likely it will reflect one of the following acid–base disorders:

Diagnostic considerations for positive and negative bicarbonate gap ($\Delta AG - \Delta CO_2$)*

Positive bicarbonate gap (> 6 mEq/L)

The serum CO_2 is reduced *less than predicted* by the change in the anion gap and suggests

a. Metabolic alkalosis and/or
b. Bicarbonate retention as compensation for respiratory acidosis

Negative bicarbonate gap (< −6 mEq/L)

The serum CO_2 is reduced *more than predicted* by the change in the anion gap and suggests

a. Hyperchloremic metabolic acidosis and/or
b. Bicarbonate excretion as compensation for respiratory alkalosis

*The more positive or negative the bicarbonate gap, the more likely there is an acid–base disturbance as described. See text for discussion.

When presented with a set of electrolytes and the possibility of an acid–base disorder, you should make the following calculations. This process may appear cumbersome at first, but it can be done quickly and without paper and pencil. After you have learned this method, I will show you a nice shortcut. The values below are from the case of the 42-year-old man presented on page 117.

1. Anion gap (AG) = $Na^+ - (Cl^- + CO_2) = 165 - (112 + 32) = 21$ mEq/L
2. ΔAG = AG − normal anion gap = 21 − 12 = 9 mEq/L

3. ΔCO_2 = normal CO_2 − measured CO_2 = 27 − 32 = −5 mEq/L
4. Bicarbonate gap = $\Delta AG - \Delta CO_2$ = 9 − (−5) = 14 mEq/L

Note that the calculations use the average normal venous CO_2 of 27 mEq/L (Fig. 7.1). It is called the *bicarbonate gap* because the bicarbonate moiety is what is buffered by organic anions; however, the serum CO_2 is used in the calculation because that is what the chemistry lab measures and what the anion gap is based on (as discussed earlier). Try not to become confused by this terminology. I purposely show the steps with *both* terms so you will understand that we are calculating the bicarbonate gap with a venous chemistry value that is usually called CO_2.

In this example, the very high bicarbonate gap of 14 mEq/L indicates a metabolic alkalosis and/or compensation for respiratory acidosis. Of course, either diagnosis is suggested even without all the calculations, because the venous CO_2 is slightly elevated; indeed, the "hidden" disturbance in this case is the metabolic acidosis, which is uncovered by calculating the AG. (Subsequent blood gas analysis showed normal $PaCO_2$, so venous CO_2 was elevated because of metabolic alkalosis.)

Shortcut to calculating the bicarbonate gap

The steps outlined above are important for understanding how the bicarbonate gap is derived and what it measures. Once you learn this method of calculation you can (and should) use the much simpler shortcut. The shortcut is derived from canceling out terms in the ΔAG and ΔCO_2 equations. Thus

$$\begin{aligned}\text{Bicarbonate gap} &= \Delta AG - \Delta CO_2 \\ &= [AG - 12] - [27 - CO_2] \\ &= [(Na^+ - Cl^- - CO_2) - 12] - [27 - CO_2] \\ &= \mathbf{Na^+ - Cl^- - 39}\end{aligned}$$

Yes, $Na^+ - Cl^- - 39$ is certainly simpler than the four separate calculations I first presented. However, I believe that you must know how to do the four steps before you can appreciate what the bicarbonate gap represents. Also, of course, the constant 39 will vary with different average values for AG and CO_2. In the following examples I calculate bicarbonate gap using both the long and short methods.

Clinical use of the bicarbonate gap

As a diagnostic aid, the bicarbonate gap is most useful when venous CO_2 is not elevated, as shown in the following case.

What are the acid–base disorders in a 28-year-old man who presents to the emergency department (ED) after several days of vomiting, nausea, and abdominal pain. His blood pressure is low, and he has tenting of the skin. He has the following electrolytes:

Na^+ = 144 mEq/L
K^+ = 4.2 mEq/L
Cl^- = 95 mEq/L
CO_2 = 14 mEq/L

1. Calculate the anion gap: $AG = Na^+ - (Cl^- + CO_2) = 144 - (95 + 14) = 35$
2. Calculate ΔAG (be sure to use the normal AG of your lab): $35 - 12 = 23$
3. Calculate ΔCO_2: $27 - 14 = 13$
4. Calculate the bicarbonate gap: $\Delta AG - \Delta CO_2 = 23 - 13 = 10$ mEq/L

Shortcut: $Na^+ - Cl^- - 39 = 144 - 95 - 39 = 10$ mEq/L

The bicarbonate gap is +10 mEq/L, indicating that the measured serum CO_2 is 10 mEq/L *higher* than expected from the ΔAG. Thus there is both an anion gap metabolic acidosis (from dehydration and poor perfusion) *and* a metabolic alkalosis (from vomiting and loss of stomach acid), but you might not appreciate the latter without calculating the bicarbonate gap. At first glance, one might just note a low CO_2 and miss the fact that it is too high for the anion gap.

Bicarbonate gap calculation can also uncover a coexisting nonanion gap metabolic acidosis, as shown in the following case.

What is (are) the acid–base disorder(s) evident in the following values, from a 27-year-old woman with acute renal failure?

Na^+ = 140 mEq/L
K^+ = 4 mEq/L
Cl^- = 115 mEq/L
CO_2 = 5 mEq/L
pH = 7.12
$PaCO_2$ = 13 mm Hg
HCO_3^- = 4 mEq/L

Clearly, the blood gases indicate a state of metabolic acidosis. But what type or types?

1. Calculate the anion gap: AG = $Na^+ - (Cl^- + CO_2) = 140 - (115 + 5) = 20$
2. Calculate ΔAG: $20 - 12 = 8$
3, Calculate ΔCO_2: $27 - 5 = 22$
4. Calculate the bicarbonate gap: $\Delta AG - \Delta CO_2 = 8 - 22 = -14$ mEq/L

Shortcut: $Na^+ - Cl^- - 39 = 140 - 115 - 39 = -14$ mEq/L

Her bicarbonate gap is significantly reduced at −14 mEq/L. Thus her measured CO_2 is 14 mEq/L *lower* than we would expect from the excess anion gap alone. Stated another way, the acid or acids causing her anion gap should have lowered venous CO_2 to only about 19 mEq/L; that her venous CO_2 is actually 5 mEq/L indicates an additional reason for the acidosis, in this case hyperchloremic metabolic acidosis. Such a situation is fairly common in patients with renal failure, who have uremia (causing elevated AG metabolic) and interstitial nephritis (causing hyperchloremic metabolic acidosis, which doesn't elevate the AG).

Clinical Problem 7.3. What is (are) the likely acid–base disorder(s) from these values?

Na^+ = 150 mEq/L
K^+ = 3.5 mEq/L
Cl^- = 102 mEq/L
CO_2 = 20 mEq/L
pH = 7.46
$PaCO_2$ = 30 mm Hg
HCO_3^- = 20 mEq/L

It bears emphasis that an abnormal bicarbonate gap doesn't diagnose with certainty the *type* of acid–base disorder. The reasoning here is the same as when confronted with just an abnormal venous CO_2 value. For example, an elevated venous CO_2 and/or positive bicarbonate gap could arise from retention of bicarbonate as compensation for respiratory acidosis. Bicarbonate retention as compensation is not considered a true metabolic alkalosis.

Likewise, a reduced venous CO_2 and/or negative bicarbonate gap could arise from bicarbonate excretion as compensation for respiratory alkalosis. Bicarbonate excretion as compensation is not considered a true metabolic acidosis. Definitions of metabolic acidosis and alkalosis are presented in Chapter 8.

Figure 7.2 presents an algorithm for using electrolytes to diagnose acid–base disorders. By following the potential paths (*arrows*), you can see that a patient can have a low venous CO_2 and still have a metabolic alkalosis. Note that mixed metabolic disorders should always be clarified by measurement of blood gases. Also, note that if AG is normal, one should not need to calculate the bicarbonate gap.

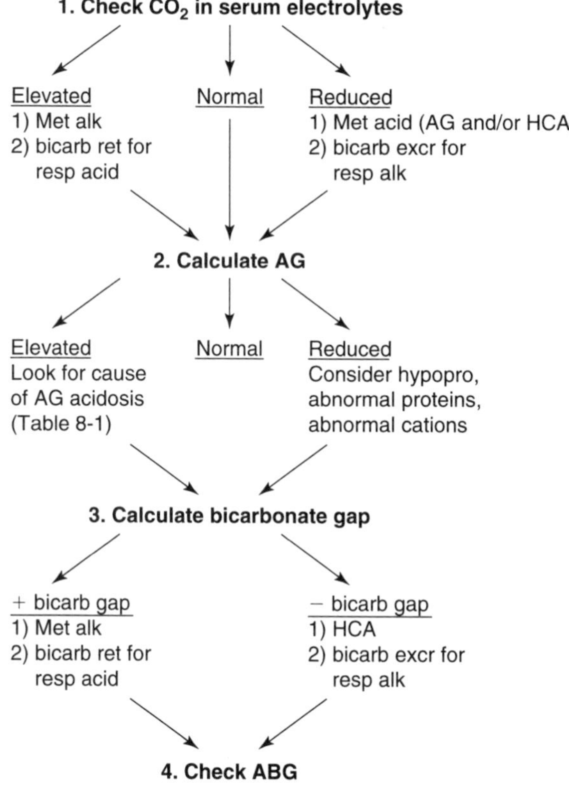

Figure 7.2. Algorithm for using electrolytes to diagnose acid–base disorders. Note that in each situation, the listed diagnoses are not mutually exclusive. See text for discussion. *Met alk,* metabolic alkalosis; *met acid,* metabolic acidosis; *HCA,* hyperchloremic acidosis; *resp alk,* respiratory alkalosis; *bicarb,* bicarbonate; *resp acid,* respiratory acidosis; *ret,* retention; *hypopro,* hypoproteinemia; *excr,* excretion.

Clinical Problem 7.4. Examine the four sets of values for AG and CO_2 and determine the acid–base disorder(s) suggested by each (choose from diagnoses a–f). Each set may be associated with more than one diagnosis. CO_2 = measured serum CO_2.

a. No evident acid–base disorder
b. AG metabolic acidosis
c. Hyperchloremic metabolic acidosis
d. Metabolic alkalosis
e. Chronic respiratory alkalosis
f. Chronic respiratory acidosis

1. AG = 22 mEq/L, CO_2 = 17 mEq/L
2. AG = 14 mEq/L, CO_2 = 17 mEq/L
3. AG = 28 mEq/L, CO_2 = 20 mEq/L
4. AG = 12 mEq/L, CO_2 = 33 mEq/L

Clinical Problem 7.5. A 47-year-old woman is brought to the ED with recent onset of fever, vomiting, and altered mental status. On examination, she appears acutely ill. Arterial blood gas values on room air are as follows.

pH = 7.42
HCO_3^- = 24 mEq/L
$PaCO_2$ = 38 mm Hg
PaO_2 = 84 mm Hg

From these values, you could reasonably conclude (one answer only):

a. There is no significant acid–base disorder involving the bicarbonate buffer system
b. The blood gases likely represent an error of measurement
c. Venous electrolytes will likely show an abnormal CO_2
d. If the patient has an acid–base disorder it must be mixed

Clinical Problem 7.6. A 34-year-old man comes to the ED complaining of increasing lethargy and swollen feet. The following laboratory values are obtained.

pH = 7.40
Na^+ = 149
$PaCO_2$ = 38 mm Hg
K^+ = 3.8
HCO_3^- = 24 mEq/L
Cl^- = 100
PaO_2 = 72 mm Hg
CO_2 = 24
BUN = 110 mg/dL
Creatinine = 8.7 mg/dL

What is(are) the acid–base disorder(s)?

BASE EXCESS VS. BICARBONATE

One of the more confusing calculations is base excess (BE). I don't use or teach BE; but because it is so often reported with blood gas values, an explanation is warranted.

Most clinicians know BE is somehow related to bicarbonate concentration, $[HCO_3^-]$, but don't know exactly how. Apart from bicarbonate, the blood contains other buffers, principally hemoglobin. When fixed acid is added to blood, the total quantity of buffer base per liter ([BB]) *decreases* in proportion to the amount of added acid, just as bicarbonate decreases. Similarly, because $[HCO_3^-]$ is part of blood's total buffer base, [BB] also *increases* in states of metabolic alkalosis. In other words, any rise or fall of $[HCO_3^-]$ will be mirrored by a rise or fall of [BB].

In theory, [BB] should more accurately assess metabolic acid–base disturbances than does $[HCO_3^-]$, because it represents all the buffer base, not just $[HCO_3^-]$. Of course, you have to know the patient's hemoglobin content to determine [BB]. When the Hb is normal at 15 g/dL, [BB] is about 48 mEq/L. When the Hb is 8 g/dL, [BB] is about 45 mEq/L.

Base excess is the difference between the patient's normal [BB] and his or her actual [BB]. Although originally based on in vitro titration of blood, and therefore a measurement, base excess as reported in blood gas labs today is actually a calculation:

$$BE = \text{normal [BB]} - \text{calculated [BB]}$$

Normally BE is zero $\pm$ 2 mEq/L. If BE has a positive value ($<$ 2 mEq/L), the patient has an excess of the metabolic component and [HCO_3^-] should also be increased. If BE has a negative value (< -2 mEq/L), the patient has a *base deficit* and [HCO_3^-] should also be decreased; sometimes this situation is referred to as *negative base excess,* an admittedly confusing term.

Base excess is a complicated way of reporting that the metabolic component of the blood—of which bicarbonate is about half the total—is increased or decreased. Because BE takes into account all the buffer base, and not just bicarbonate, there is not a 1:1, or exact linear, relationship between BE and bicarbonate.

The following data on one sample of arterial blood include both bicarbonate and base excess. The BE of 15 mEq/L indicates a large increase in the metabolic component; this is also reflected in the calculated bicarbonate, which is 18 mEq/L above normal. Either value, *along with the pH and $PaCO_2$,* suggests two acid–base disorders: metabolic alkalosis and compensated respiratory acidosis.

pH	7.45
SaO_2	93%
$PaCO_2$	62 mm Hg
Hb	13.9 g/dL
PaO_2	73 mm Hg
BE	15 mEq/L
HCO_3^-	42 mEq/L

There are four reasons why I don't use base excess in blood gas interpretation.

1. The terminology is confusing, particularly when BE is negative and one hears the term *negative base excess.*
2. BE is a calculation, the equation for which may vary from lab to lab (some labs calculate BE for whole blood only, whereas other labs calculate BE for all the extracellular fluid). The formula is complicated and nothing any clinician needs to know, unlike the formulas for oxygen content or anion gap, for example. BE thus adds a layer of mysticism (where did this number come from?) and complexity to blood gas interpretation.
3. In chronic respiratory disorders, where increases or decreases in HCO_3^-

may be appropriate, the abnormal BE may suggest a metabolic problem that requires attention. For example, the values pH = 7.36, $PaCO_2$ = 58 mm Hg, and HCO_3^- = 34 mEq/L may represent a patient's steady state of chronic respiratory acidosis; a BE of 12 mEq/L reported with these data suggests significant metabolic abnormality, when in fact the metabolic response—renal retention of bicarbonate for compensation of respiratory acidosis—is desired and appropriate.

4. By closely examining the calculated bicarbonate value, blood gases can be adequately interpreted without knowing the BE. Because not all labs report BE, but do calculate HCO_3^-, the clinician should become thoroughly familiar with interpreting acid–base status without BE. Facility in using the HCO_3^- value should eliminate the need for calculating or worrying about base excess.

In summary, BE is a calculation based on the concept of how much the total base for the blood sample varies from the normal value; the result could be a positive or negative number (the latter is called negative base excess or base deficit). BE does not take into account the appropriateness of the excess or deficit and provides no more useful information than is provided by the calculated bicarbonate value. For these reasons, BE is not used to interpret blood gases in this book.

ANSWERS TO CLINICAL PROBLEMS

7.1. There is a 10 mEq/L discrepancy between the calculated arterial HCO_3^- (34 mEq/L) and measured venous CO_2 (24 mEq/L). If pH and $PaCO_2$ are correct, so is the calculated HCO_3^-, and you must discard the venous CO_2 as inaccurate. Of course, either the pH or $PaCO_2$ could be measured incorrectly, and then the calculated HCO_3^- would also be incorrect. But if you are going to interpret the data as presented, you must accept *either* the blood gas data or the venous CO_2—not both. The blood gas values certainly suggest a state of metabolic alkalosis (elevated HCO_3^-). Possible reasons for differences between calculated arterial HCO_3^- and measured venous CO_2 are listed in Table 7.2.

7.2. Assume the venous CO_2 and the arterial HCO_3^- are equal. Calculate the venous CO_2:

Anion gap = $Na^+ - (Cl^- + CO_2)$ = 20 mEq/L
Since 20 mEq/L = 145 − (104 + CO_2)
Then CO_2 = 21 mEq/L

You can now calculate pH from the H–H equation.

$$pH = 6.1 + \log \frac{21}{0.03(50)} = 7.25$$

7.3.

1. Calculate the anion gap: AG = $Na^+ - (Cl^- + CO_2) = 150 - (102 + 20) = 28$
2. Calculate ΔAG: $28 - 12 = 16$
3. Calculate ΔCO_2: $27 - 20 = 7$
4. Calculate the bicarbonate gap: $\Delta AG - \Delta CO_2 = 16 - 7 = 9$ mEq/L

Shortcut: $Na^+ - Cl^- - 39 = 150 - 102 - 39 = 9$ mEq/L

In this example, the AG increased by 9 mEq/L more than the serum CO_2 fell, making the measured CO_2 higher than expected; thus there is likely a co-existing *metabolic alkalosis.* In other words, even though there is an increased anion gap *and* a lower than normal venous CO_2 value, the patient *also* has a metabolic alkalosis. Finally, the patient also has respiratory alkalosis.

From the blood gases alone, without looking at the electrolytes, you would be able to diagnose only respiratory alkalosis. And by calculating just the anion gap (without checking the bicarbonate gap), you would likely miss the fact that there are both an anion gap metabolic acidosis *and* a metabolic alkalosis in this patient. Such situations—combined metabolic acidosis and alkalosis—are more common than you may realize, particularly in alcoholics and in patients with renal disease. An example would be a patient who has been vomiting for several days (metabolic alkalosis) and who then develops hypotension (causing lactic acidosis).

7.4. The diagnoses (Dx) given are not mutually exclusive and may coexist. Arterial blood gases and a full clinical assessment would be necessary to make complete diagnoses.

1.

ΔAG	= 10
ΔCO_2	= 10
Bicarbonate gap	= 0
Dx	= b

2.

ΔAG	= 2
ΔCO_2	= 10
Bicarbonate gap	= −8
Dx	= c, e

3.

ΔAG	= 16
ΔCO_2	= 7
Bicarbonate gap	= 9
Dx	= b, d, f

4.

ΔAG	= 0
ΔCO_2	= −6
Bicarbonate gap	= 6
Dx	= d, f

7.5. d. If the patient has an acid–base disorder it must be mixed. Answer a is incorrect, because a normal HCO_3^- does not rule out an acid–base disorder involving the bicarbonate buffer system; there can be two or more disorders (i.e., metabolic alkalosis and metabolic acidosis) that balance out to give a normal bicarbonate. Answer b is incorrect, because there is no basis for assuming an error of measurement from the information provided. Answer c is incorrect, because the venous CO_2 should be close to the calculated arterial HCO_3^-. Answer d is correct for the same reason that answer a is incorrect. This patient presented with a mixed acid–base disorder. Further information about her lab values is provided in the next problem.

7.6. First, note that pH, PCO_2, calculated HCO_3^-, and serum CO_2 are all normal (and, in this case, the venous CO_2 = the arterial HCO_3^-). At first glance, it appears there is no acid–base disorder and that the only obvious abnormality is the markedly elevated BUN and creatinine. By going through the steps outlined in this answer, however, a more complete picture emerges.

1. Calculate the anion gap: $AG = Na^+ - (Cl^- + CO_2) = 149 - (100 + 24) = 25$
2. Calculate ΔAG: $25 - 12 = 13$
3. Calculate ΔCO_2: $27 - 24 = 3$
4. Calculate the bicarbonate gap: $13 - 3 = 10$

Shortcut: $Na^+ - Cl^- - 39 = 149 - 100 - 39 = 10$ mEq/L

The bicarbonate gap of +10 mEq/L indicates a metabolic alkalosis. Thus this patient, with normal pH and $PaCO_2$, has both metabolic acidosis and metabolic alkalosis. The patient was both uremic (causing metabolic acidosis) and had been taking a diuretic (metabolic alkalosis).

CHAPTER

8

Primary and Mixed Acid–Base Disorders

RELATIONSHIPS AMONG THE H–H VARIABLES

The simple relationship of pH to the HCO_3^-:$PaCO_2$ ratio can be used to describe the four primary acid–base disorders and their compensatory changes (Fig. 8.1). In describing any acid–base disorder, a distinction should be made between changes in the blood and the changes in the patient; the former go by the terms *acidemia* and *alkalemia,* the latter by the terms *acidosis* and *alkalosis* (Winters 1965). The reason for this important distinction will become clearer when we discuss mixed acid–base disorders. Some important definitions are given below.

Acidemia. Present when blood pH < 7.35.

Acidosis. A primary physiologic process that, occurring alone, tends to cause acidemia. Examples include metabolic acidosis from low-perfusion lactic acidosis and respiratory acidosis from acute hypoventilation. If the patient has an alkalosis at the same time, the resulting blood pH may be low, normal, or high.

Alkalemia. Present when blood pH > 7.45.

Alkalosis. A primary physiologic process that, occurring alone, tends to cause alkalemia. Examples include metabolic alkalosis from excessive diuretic therapy and respiratory alkalosis from acute hyperventilation. If the patient has an acidosis at the same time, the resulting blood pH may be high, normal, or low.

Primary acid–base disorder. One of the four acid–base disturbances manifested by an initial change in either HCO_3^- or $PaCO_2$ (Fig. 8.1). If HCO_3^- is first to change, the disorder is either a metabolic acidosis (reduced HCO_3^-, acidemia) or metabolic alkalosis (elevated HCO_3^-, alkalemia). If the $PaCO_2$ is first to change, the problem is either respiratory alkalosis (reduced $PaCO_2$, alkalemia) or respiratory acidosis (elevated $PaCO_2$, acidemia).

Compensation. The change in HCO_3^- or $PaCO_2$ that occurs as a result of the primary event. *Compensatory changes are not classified by the terms*

PRIMARY EVENT | COMPENSATORY EVENT

Metabolic acidosis

$$\downarrow pH \cong \frac{\downarrow HCO_3^-}{PaCO_2} \qquad \downarrow pH \cong \frac{\downarrow HCO_3^-}{\downarrow PaCO_2}$$

Metabolic alkalosis

$$\uparrow pH \cong \frac{\uparrow HCO_3^-}{PaCO_2} \qquad \uparrow pH \cong \frac{\uparrow HCO_3^-}{\uparrow PaCO_2}$$

Respiratory acidosis

$$\downarrow pH \cong \frac{HCO_3^-\,*}{\uparrow PaCO_2} \qquad \downarrow pH \cong \frac{\uparrow HCO_3^-}{\uparrow PaCO_2}$$

Respiratory alkalosis

$$\uparrow pH \cong \frac{HCO_3^-\,**}{\downarrow PaCO_2} \qquad \uparrow pH \cong \frac{\downarrow HCO_3^-}{\downarrow PaCO_2}$$

Figure 8.1. The four primary acid–base disorders and their compensatory changes. The primary event leads to a large change in pH (*large arrows*). Compensation—changes in HCO_3^- and $PaCO_2$ (*small arrows*)—attempts to normalize the HCO_3^-:$PaCO_2$ ratio and bring the pH back toward normal (*small arrows*). Each primary disorder may be caused by a variety of specific clinical conditions (Table 8.1).

* For each 10 mm Hg increase in $PaCO_2$, HCO_3^- increases by ~ 1 mEq/L due to biochemical buffering. See text for discussion.

** For each 10 mm Hg decrease in $PaCO_2$, HCO_3^- decreases by ~ 2 mEq/L due to biochemical buffering. See text for discussion.

acidosis and alkalosis. For example, a patient who hyperventilates (lowers $PaCO_2$) solely as compensation for metabolic acidosis does *not* have a respiratory alkalosis. Because the hyperventilation occurs solely as compensation for metabolic acidosis there is no respiratory alkalosis, the latter being a primary disorder that, alone, would lead to alkalemia. In uncomplicated metabolic acidosis the patient will never develop alkalemia.

TABLE 8.1. SOME CLINICAL CAUSES OF THE FOUR PRIMARY ACID–BASE DISORDERS

Metabolic acidosis
- With increased anion gap
  - Lactic acidosis, ketoacidosis, poisoning and overdose (e.g., paraldehyde, ethylene glycol, methanol, aspirin)
- With normal anion gap
  - Diarrhea, renal tubular acidosis, interstitial nephritis, excess NH_4Cl administration, drainage from a ureterosigmoidostomy, acetazolamide administration

Metabolic alkalosis
- Chloride-responsive (responds to NaCl or KCl)
  - Contraction alkalosis, diuretics, corticosteroids, gastric suctioning, vomiting
- Chloride-resistant
  - Any hyperaldosterone state (e.g., Cushing's syndrome; Bartter's syndrome), severe K^+ depletion

Respiratory acidosis (respiratory failure)
- Central nervous system depression
  - Drug overdose, anesthesia
- Chest bellows weakness or dysfunction
  - Myasthenia gravis, polio, massive obesity, diaphragm paralysis, flail chest, paralyzing agents
- Disease of lungs and/or upper airway
  - Severe asthma attack, chronic obstructive pulmonary disease, severe pneumonia, severe pulmonary edema, upper airway obstruction

Respiratory alkalosis
- Voluntary hyperventilation
- Hypoxemia (includes altitude)
- Liver failure
- Anxiety hyperventilation syndrome
- Sepsis
- Any acute pulmonary problem
  - Acute pulmonary embolism, pneumonia, mild asthma attack, mild pulmonary edema

Clinical Problem 8.1. For each of the following situations, indicate which of the four primary acid–base disorders is present and give the nature and direction of compensation (e.g., $\uparrow HCO_3^-$). Answer without consulting Figure 8.1.

	CONDITIONS		PRIMARY DISORDER	COMPENSATION
a.	↓pH	↓HCO_3^-		
b.	↓pH	↑$PaCO_2$		
c.	↑pH	↓$PaCO_2$		
d.	↑pH	↑HCO_3^-		

THE FOUR PRIMARY ACID–BASE DISORDERS AND THEIR CLINICAL CAUSES

The diagnosis of any primary acid–base disorder is analogous to diagnoses like anemia and fever; a specific cause must be sought to provide proper treatment. Each primary acid–base disorder (Fig. 8.1) arises from one or more specific clinical conditions, although the specific clinical cause may not be readily apparent. Table 8.1 lists the most common clinical conditions that lead to acid–base disturbances.

Respiratory alkalosis and respiratory acidosis

Any discussion of primary acid–base disorders should begin with respiratory alkalosis and acidosis. Together, these two disorders characterize the body's "titration" of carbon dioxide. Table 8.2 shows the changes in HCO_3^- and pH as $PaCO_2$ rises from 15 to 90 mm Hg. These data, generated experimentally on human subjects in two separate studies (Arbus et al. 1969; Brackett et al. 1965), are also graphed on the acid–base map as the bands for acute respiratory alkalosis and acidosis (Fig. 8.2).

For the low $PaCO_2$ band (acute respiratory alkalosis), subjects were hyperventilated during anesthesia for elective surgery; their arterial blood gases were measured within 10 min. For the high $PaCO_2$ band (acute respiratory acidosis), healthy volunteers were placed in an environmental chamber and given 5% CO_2 to inhale; their blood gases were also measured within 10 min.

The CO_2 titration band is especially useful in the presence of mixed acid–base disorders. Respiratory disorders with blood gas values falling outside the band indicate that the problem is not acute or that the problem may be mixed.

Clinical Problem 8.2. A patient's arterial blood gas shows pH = 7.14, $PaCO_2$ = 70 mm Hg, and HCO_3^- = 23 mEq/L. How would you describe the likely acid–base disorder(s)?

TABLE 8.2. CHANGES IN PH AND HCO_3^- WITH ACUTE CHANGES IN $PACO_2$.

Data for each $PaCO_2$ value represent the 95% confidence limits for pH and bicarbonate when $PaCO_2$ changes acutely (before any renal compensation takes place): 95% of all subjects with acute hyperventilation or hypoventilation, to the degree shown and with no other acid–base disorder, should have blood gas values within these ranges. Note that bicarbonate decreases with acute hyperventilation and increases with acute hypoventilation. These data are graphed in Figure 8.2 as the bands for acute respiratory alkalosis and acidosis.

$PaCO_2$ (mm Hg)	pH	HCO_3^- (mEq/L)
15	7.61–7.74	15.3–20.5
20	7.55–7.66	17.7–22.8
30	7.45–7.53	21.0–25.6
40	7.38–7.45	22.8–26.8
50	7.31–7.36	24.1–27.5
60	7.24–7.29	25.1–27.9
70	7.19–7.23	25.7–28.5
80	7.14–7.18	26.2–28.9
90	7.09–7.13	26.5–29.2

Data from Brackett NC Jr, Cohen JJ, Schwartz WB. Carbon dioxide titration curve of normal man. N Engl J Med 1965;272:6–12; and Arbus GS, Hebert LA, Levesque PR, et al. Characterization and clinical application of the "significance band" for acute respiratory alkalosis. N Engl J Med 1969;280:117–123.

Metabolic acidosis

Metabolic acidosis is conveniently divided into increased and normal anion gap acidosis (Table 8.1). Increased anion gap acidosis arises when excess acid that has an unmeasured anion is added to the blood (e.g., lactic acidosis: lactate anion). Normal AG acidosis arises when chloride, which is routinely measured, is added to the blood (e.g., NH_4Cl administration) or when there is a loss of bicarbonate from the blood (e.g., profuse diarrhea, renal tubular acidosis) that is replaced by chloride.

The expected human compensation (95% confidence band) for metabolic acidosis is shown in Figure 8.2. This band was generated from data on patients with uncomplicated metabolic acidosis (e.g., diabetic ketoacidosis) who had been in this state for at least 24 h (Asch et al. 1969; Pierce et al. 1970). Any patient with metabolic acidosis whose blood gas values fall outside this band likely has either very early metabolic acidosis (before full compensation has taken place) or a mixed acid–base disorder.

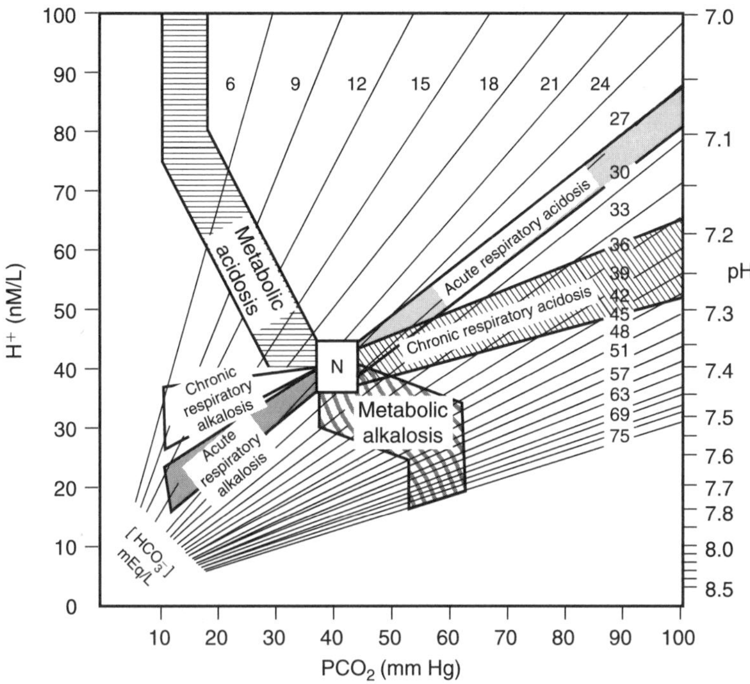

Figure 8.2. Acid–base map showing confidence bands for the four primary acid–base disorders, plus the bands for chronic respiratory acidosis and chronic respiratory alkalosis. Human titration curve for carbon dioxide is a continuous band made by joining the bands for acute respiratory alkalosis ($PaCO_2$ from 10 to 40 mm Hg) and acidosis ($PaCO_2$ from 40 to 100 mm Hg); see also Table 8.2. Reprinted with permission from Goldberg M, Green SB, Moss ML, et al. Computer-based instruction and diagnosis of acid–base disorders. JAMA 1973;223:269–275.

Metabolic alkalosis

Metabolic alkalosis can occur from excess bicarbonate added to the blood or from loss of HCl. Excess bicarbonate can occur from exogenous administration or from excess renal reabsorption (as seen with diuretic therapy). Loss of HCl is commonly seen with nasogastric suctioning and vomiting.

Unlike the other primary acid–base disorders, there is no narrow confidence band for metabolic alkalosis; the one shown in Figure 8.2 encompasses both normal and high $PaCO_2$ values. The degree of change in $PaCO_2$ as compensation for pure metabolic alkalosis is wide ranging. Studies have actually described two broad compensation bands for this disorder, depending on the degree of bicarbonate elevation (Javaheri 1982; Javaheri & Kazemi 1987).

DOES THE PATIENT HAVE A MIXED ACID–BASE DISORDER?

There is perhaps no more confusing topic related to blood gases than mixed acid–base disorders. This topic was discussed in Chapter 7 in regard to the serum electrolytes. As was pointed out, calculation of the anion and bicarbonate gaps can help uncover mixed *metabolic* disorders (e.g., anion gap metabolic acidosis and metabolic alkalosis). Of course, to accurately diagnose the specific disorders and their relative severity at least one set of blood gases is usually necessary.

Once blood gases are available, acid–base maps, such as the one in Figure 8.2, are often brought out to help unravel mixed disorders. These maps are helpful *if* readily available and used properly, which are not always the case. In fact, the clinical history plus basic blood gas and electrolyte data, when closely examined, are often sufficient to figure out most mixed disorders, because specific changes for pH, $PaCO_2$, and HCO_3^- in single acid–base disorders, except for metabolic alkalosis, occur in a fairly predictable fashion. When there is significant deviation from the expected changes, a mixed disorder is usually present. I have found the following four tips especially helpful in diagnosing mixed acid–base disorders.

TIP 1. Don't interpret any blood gas data for acid–base diagnosis without also examining the corresponding serum electrolytes. Remember that a serum CO_2 out of the normal range always represents some type of acid–base disorder (barring lab or transcription error) and that serum CO_2 may be normal in the presence of two or more acid–base disorders. Calculate the anion gap (AG); if it is elevated, calculate the bicarbonate gap. An AG $\geq$ 20 mEq/L strongly indicates an anion gap acidosis. If the bicarbonate gap deviates more than $\pm$ 6 mEq/L, there is likely another acid–base disorder besides AG metabolic acidosis (see Chapter 7, including Figure 7.2).

TIP 2. Single acid–base disorders do not lead to normal blood pH. Although pH can end up in the normal range (7.35–7.45) with single disorders of a mild degree, a truly normal pH with distinctly abnormal HCO_3^- and $PaCO_2$ invariably suggests two or more primary disorders. For example, you may find pH = 7.40, $PaCO_2$ = 20 mm Hg, and HCO_3^- = 12 mEq/L in a patient with sepsis. This patient's normal pH resulted from two coexisting and unstable acid–base disorders: acute respiratory alkalosis and metabolic acidosis.

TIP 3. Simplified rules predict the pH and HCO_3^- for a given change in $PaCO_2$. If the pH or HCO_3^- is higher or lower than expected for the change in $PaCO_2$, the patient probably has a metabolic acid–base disorder as well. The rules in Table 8.3 show the expected changes in pH and HCO_3^- for *a 10 mm Hg change* in $PaCO_2$ from either primary hypoventilation (respiratory acidosis) or primary hyperventilation (respiratory alkalosis).

The rules in Table 8.3 are quite useful in diagnosing a mixed acid–base disorder when there is respiratory acidosis or respiratory alkalosis. These two conditions, of course, describe acute changes in $PaCO_2$ and, therefore, acute changes in the dissolved CO_2 in the blood. Changes in $PaCO_2$, i.e., in the dissolved fraction of CO_2, affect the hydration of dissolved CO_2 with H_2O, which is a reversible reaction:

$$CO_2 + H_2O \leftrightarrow H_2CO_3 \leftrightarrow H^+ + HCO_3^-$$

Acute CO_2 retention (i.e., acute respiratory acidosis) drives the hydration reaction more to the *right* than normal; as a result, HCO_3^- *increases* slightly. Acute CO_2 excretion (i.e., acute respiratory alkalosis) drives the hydration reaction more to the *left* than normal, and HCO_3^- *decreases* slightly. These changes in HCO_3^- are instantaneous by virtue of changes in the CO_2 hydration reaction and have *nothing* to do with the kidneys or renal compensation. Thus

1. A normal or slightly low HCO_3^- in the presence of hypercapnia suggests a concomitant *metabolic acidosis,* e.g., pH = 7.27, $PaCO_2$ = 50 mm Hg, and HCO_3^- = 22 mEq/L.
2. A normal or slightly elevated HCO_3^- in the presence of hypocapnia suggests a concomitant *metabolic alkalosis,* e.g., pH = 7.56, $PaCO_2$ = 30 mm Hg, and HCO_3^- = 26 mEq/L.

TIP 4. In maximally compensated metabolic acidosis (which takes 12–24 h), the following formula applies:

TABLE 8.3. CHANGES IN pH AND HCO_3^- FOR A 10 mm Hg CHANGE IN $PaCO_2$

CONDITION	ACUTE	CHRONIC
Respiratory acidosis ($PaCO_2$ up to 70 mm Hg)	pH down by 0.07 HCO_3^- up by 1 mEq/L	pH down by 0.03 HCO_3^- up by 3–4 mEq/L
Respiratory alkalosis ($PaCO_2$ down to 20 mm Hg)	pH up by 0.08 HCO_3^- down by 2 mEq/L	pH up by 0.03 HCO_3^- down by 5 mEq/L

$$\text{Expected PaCO}_2 = (1.5 \times \text{serum CO}_2) + (8 \pm 2)$$

A shortcut to this formula is the interesting observation, in maximally compensated metabolic acidosis, that the numerical value of $PaCO_2$ should be the same (or close to) the last two digits of arterial pH (Narins 1980). Thus:

$$\text{Expected PaCO}_2 = \text{last two digits of pH} \pm 2$$

In contrast, the compensation for metabolic alkalosis (by increasing $PaCO_2$) is highly variable, and in some cases there may be no or minimal compensation.

For each of the following sets of arterial blood gas values, what is(are) the likely acid–base disorder(s)?

a. pH = 7.28, $PaCO_2$ = 50 mm Hg, HCO_3^- = 23 mEq/L
b. pH = 7.50, $PaCO_2$ = 33 mm Hg, HCO_3^- = 25 mEq/L
c. pH = 7.25, $PaCO_2$ = 30 mm Hg, HCO_3^- = 14 mEq/L

In case a, the bicarbonate is lower than expected for acute hypoventilation; the patient has respiratory acidosis *and* metabolic acidosis. In case b, bicarbonate is higher than expected for acute hyperventilation; the patient has respiratory alkalosis *and* metabolic alkalosis. In case c, $PaCO_2$ is higher than expected for fully compensated metabolic acidosis, suggesting a concomitant respiratory disorder or very early metabolic acidosis.

Always keep in mind that *any* isolated measurement of pH and $PaCO_2$ can be explained by two or more co-existing acid–base disorders. Thus, even when blood gas values fall into one of the 95% confidence bands, the patient *may still* have a mixed disorder. Often, the only way to know for sure is by detailed analysis of all the clinical and laboratory information and close patient follow up.

Explain the acid–base status of a 35-year-old man with the following lab values, who was admitted to hospital with pneumonia.

pH = 7.52	PaO_2 = 62 mm Hg
Na^+ = 145 mEq/L	K^+ = 2.9 mEq/L

$PaCO_2 = 30$ mm Hg $CO_2 = 21$ mEq/L
$Cl^- = 98$ mEq/L

His pH and $PaCO_2$ fit into the band of acute respiratory alkalosis. He has moderate hypoxemia, and the blood gas data alone could be explained by acute hyperventilation owing to pneumonia. But the anion gap is elevated at 26 mEq/L, indicating a concomitant metabolic acidosis. The ΔAG is 14 mEq/L, giving an expected serum CO_2 of 13 mEq/L and a bicarbonate gap of +8 mEq/L. Thus the patient manifests *three separate* acid–base disorders: respiratory alkalosis (from pneumonia), metabolic acidosis (from renal disease), and hypokalemic metabolic alkalosis (from excessive diuretic therapy). The result of all this acid–base abnormality? Blood gas values that are indistinguishable from those of simple acute respiratory alkalosis.

SUMMARY—CLINICAL AND LABORATORY APPROACH TO ACID–BASE DIAGNOSIS

Each primary acid–base disorder should be viewed as a physiologic process caused by a specific clinical condition or disease, not simply as changes in blood gas and electrolyte values. This view allows for unraveling complex or mixed acid–base disorders. Points to remember for proper acid–base diagnosis and management can be summarized as follows (Fig. 8.3).

- Determine existence of an acid–base disorder from arterial blood gas and/or serum electrolyte measurements. For electrolytes, follow the steps outlined in Figure 7.2. Check the serum CO_2 for an abnormal value. Calculate the AG; and if elevated, calculate the bicarbonate gap.
- If the measured pH and/or $PaCO_2$ are abnormal, you should be able to discern at least one primary acid–base disorder from the observed changes (Fig. 8.1). The changes for each primary disorder are straightforward and should be committed to memory.
- Examine the pH, $PaCO_2$, and HCO_3^- for deviations that may indicate mixed acid–base disorders (Tips 2–4 and Table 8.3).
- Use a full clinical assessment (history; physical exam; other lab data, including previous arterial blood gases and serum electrolytes) to explain each acid–base disorder (Table 8.1). Remember that coexisting clinical conditions may lead to opposing acid disorders, so that pH can be high when there is an obvious acidosis or low when there is an obvious alkalosis.

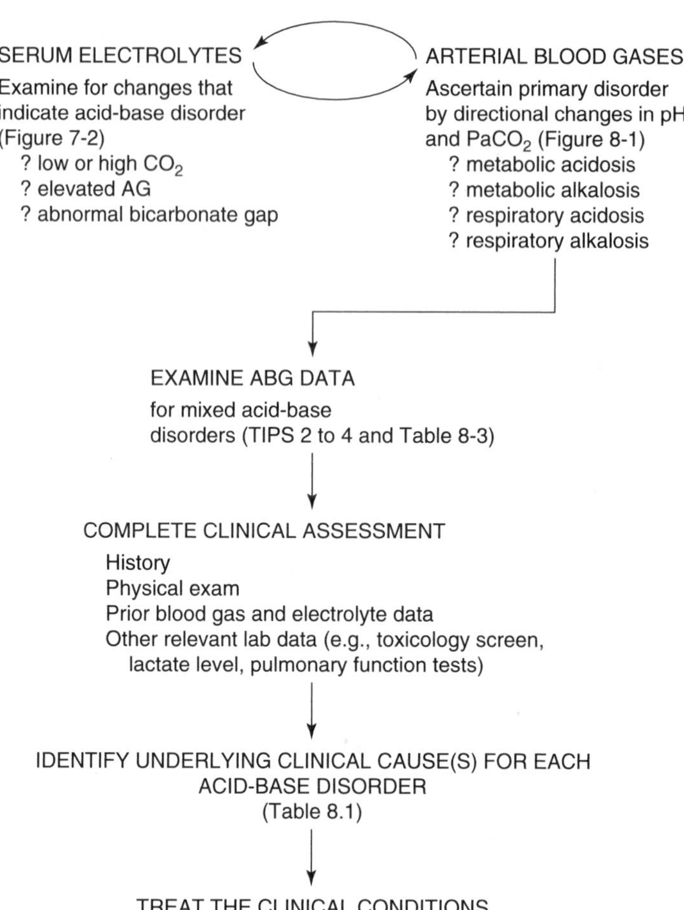

Figure 8.3. Clinical approach to the diagnosis of simple and complex acid–base disorders. See text for discussion.

- Treat the underlying clinical condition(s); this will usually suffice to correct most acid–base disorders. If there is concern that acidemia or alkalemia is life-threatening, aim toward correcting the pH into the range of 7.30–7.52 ([H^+] 50–30 nM/L).
- Clinical judgment should always apply. See Pitfalls 12–14 outlined in Chapter 13.

Clinical Problem 8.3. A 45-year-old man comes to hospital complaining of dyspnea for 3 days. Arterial blood gas reveals pH = 7.35, $PaCO_2$ = 60 mm Hg, PaO_2 = 57 mm Hg, and HCO_3^- = 31 mEq/L. How would you characterize his acid–base status?

Clinical Problem 8–4. A 53-year-old man initially presents to the emergency department with the following blood gas values:

FIO_2 = 0.21
PaO_2 = 40 mm Hg
pH = 7.51
HCO_3^- = 39 mEq/L
$PaCO_2$ = 50 mm Hg

At this point his acid–base disorder is *best* characterized as:

a. Metabolic alkalosis alone
b. Metabolic alkalosis plus respiratory acidosis
c. Respiratory acidosis with metabolic compensation
d. Can't be certain without more information

He is found to have congestive heart failure and is treated with supplemental oxygen and diuretics. Three days later he is clinically improved, with pH = 7.38, $PaCO_2$ = 60 mm Hg, HCO_3^- = 34 mEq/L, and PaO_2 = 73 mm Hg (on FIO_2 = 24%). How would you characterize his acid–base status now?

Clinical Problem 8.5. The following values are found in a 65-year-old patient.

ARTERIAL BLOOD GASES		VENOUS BLOOD MEASUREMENTS	
MEASURE	VALUE	MEASURE	VALUE
pH	7.51	Na^+	155 mEq/L
$PaCO_2$	50 mm Hg	K^+	5.5 mEq/L
HCO_3^-	39 mEq/L	Cl^-	90 mEq/L

ARTERIAL BLOOD GASES		VENOUS BLOOD MEASUREMENTS	
MEASURE	VALUE	MEASURE	VALUE
		CO_2	40 mEq/L
		BUN	121 mg/dL
		Glucose	77 mg/dL

Which of the following most closely describes this patient's acid–base status?

a. Severe metabolic acidosis
b. Severe respiratory acidosis
c. Respiratory acidosis plus metabolic alkalosis
d. Metabolic alkalosis plus metabolic acidosis
e. Respiratory acidosis plus respiratory alkalosis

Clinical Problem 8.6. A 52-year-old woman has been mechanically ventilated for 2 days following a drug overdose. Her arterial blood gas values and electrolytes, stable for the past 12 h, show

pH = 7.45
Na^+ = 142 mEq/L
$PaCO_2$ = 25 mm Hg
K^+ = 4.0 mEq/L
Cl^- = 100 mEq/L
CO_2 = 18 mEq/L

Based on this information, how would you assess her acid–base status?

Clinical Problem 8.7. An 18-year-old college student is admitted to the ICU for an acute asthma attack, after not responding to treatment received in the emergency department. ABG values (on room air) show pH = 7.46, $PaCO_2$ = 25 mm Hg, HCO_3^- = 17 mEq/L, PaO_2 = 55 mm Hg, and SaO_2 = 87%. Her peak expiratory flow rate is 95 L/min (25% of predicted value). Asthma medication is continued. Two hours later she becomes more tired, and peak flow is < 60 L/min. Blood gas values (on 40% oxygen) now show pH = 7.20, $PaCO_2$ = 52 mm Hg, HCO_3^- = 20 mEq/L, and PaO_2 = 65 mm Hg. At this point intubation and mechanical ventilation are considered. What is her acid–base status?

Clinical Problem 8.8. A 72-year-old man is admitted in shock, with 70 mm Hg systolic blood pressure. He has a history of chronic obstructive pulmonary disease, and his baseline ABG is pH = 7.34, $PaCO_2$ = 68 mm Hg, PaO_2 = 65 mm Hg (on supplemental oxygen), and HCO_3^- = 36 mEq/L. He takes medication for a heart condition. Initial arterial blood gas results on admission (FIO_2 = 0.40) show

pH = 7.10
PaO_2 = 35 mm Hg
$PaCO_2$ = 70 mm Hg
SaO_2 = 58%
HCO_3^- = 21 mEq/L

He is intubated. Repeat blood gases (on the same FIO_2) show

pH = 7.30
PaO_2 = 87 mm Hg
$PaCO_2$ = 40 mm Hg
SaO_2 = 98%
HCO_3^- = 19 mEq/L

Assuming his anion gap is elevated at 23 mEq/L, how would you described the acid–base changes?

Clinical Problem 8.9. To review, state whether each of the following statements is true or false.

a. Metabolic acidosis is always present when the measured serum CO_2 changes acutely from 24 to 21 mEq/L.
b. In acute respiratory acidosis, bicarbonate initially rises because of

the reaction of CO_2 with water and the resultant formation of H_2CO_3.

c. If pH and $PaCO_2$ are both above normal, the calculated bicarbonate must also be above normal.
d. An abnormal serum CO_2 value always indicates an acid–base disorder of some type.
e. The compensation for chronic elevation of $PaCO_2$ is renal excretion of bicarbonate.
f. A normal pH with abnormal HCO_3^- or $PaCO_2$ suggests the presence of two or more acid–base disorders.
g. A normal serum CO_2 value indicates there is no acid–base disorder.
h. Normal arterial blood gas values rule out the presence of an acid–base disorder.

ANSWERS TO CLINICAL PROBLEMS

8.1.

	CONDITIONS		PRIMARY DISORDER	COMPENSATION
a.	↓pH	↓HCO_3^-	Metabolic acidosis	↓$PaCO_2$
b.	↓pH	↑$PaCO_2$	Respiratory acidosis	↑HCO_3^-
c.	↑pH	↓$PaCO_2$	Respiratory alkalosis	↓HCO_3^-
d.	↑pH	↑HCO_3^-	Metabolic alkalosis	↑$PaCO_2$

8.2. Acute elevation of $PaCO_2$ leads to reduced pH, i.e., an acute respiratory acidosis. However, is the problem *only* acute respiratory acidosis or is there some additional process? For every 10 mm Hg rise in $PaCO_2$ (before any renal compensation), pH falls about 0.07 units. Because this patient's pH is down 0.26, or 0.05 more than expected for a 30 mm Hg increase in $PaCO_2$, there must be an additional metabolic problem.

Another way to approach this problem is to examine the calculated HCO_3^-; it is low normal. With acute CO_2 retention of this degree, the HCO_3^- should be *elevated* 3 mEq/L. Thus a low-normal HCO_3^- with increased $PaCO_2$ is another way to uncover an additional metabolic disorder. Decreased vascular perfusion leading to mild lactic acidosis would explain the metabolic component.

8.3. The $PaCO_2$ and HCO_3^- are elevated, but HCO_3^- is elevated more than would be expected from acute respiratory acidosis. Because the patient has been dyspneic for several days, it is fair to assume a chronic acid–base disorder. Most likely this patient has a chronic or partially compensated respiratory acidosis. Without electrolyte data and more history, you cannot diagnose an accompanying metabolic disorder.

8.4. Here the answer must be d. If an acid–base disorder is found (from blood gas, electrolyte data), the next logical step is to determine the clinical causes(s). An elevated $PaCO_2$, pH, and HCO_3^- certainly suggest a metabolic alkalosis, but there are other possibilities. Isolated blood gas values should be viewed as a single point on a plot that can be arrived at from various pathways and not as diagnostic of any particular acid–base disorder. Making a diagnosis of "metabolic alkalosis" solely on the basis of blood gas values has two potential pitfalls.

Pitfall 1. It suggests a final diagnosis, which is not the case. There are several causes of metabolic alkalosis and the *clinical reason* must be found and corrected. *Acidosis* and *alkalosis,* with their adjectives *metabolic* and *respiratory,* are analogous to "anemia" or "fever." Acidosis and alkalosis should always be viewed as manifestations of underlying clinical problems and never as clinical diagnoses in themselves.

Pitfall 2. The patient may *not* have metabolic alkalosis or may have metabolic alkalosis *plus* another serious acid–base disorder. In fact, this patient's initial blood gas values represent several clinical possibilities: uncomplicated metabolic alkalosis, chronic respiratory acidosis followed by acute hyperventilation (acute respiratory alkalosis), and respiratory acidosis complicated by metabolic alkalosis. For example, suppose the patient's pulmonary function tests and blood gas values were normal 1 week earlier, and in the interval he had taken diuretics; a *primary metabolic alkalosis* would then be the most likely diagnosis. On the other hand, he could be a patient with chronic CO_2 retention (e.g., $PaCO_2$ = 60 mm Hg and pH = 7.41); he then develops pneumonia and hyperventilates, lowering the $PaCO_2$ from 60 to 50 mm Hg and raising the pH above normal. This last situation would reflect a state of chronic respiratory acidosis plus an acute increase in ventilation (respiratory alkalosis), not a primary metabolic alkalosis. Thus the patient could have an isolated metabolic problem, an isolated respiratory problem, or a combination. Only by a detailed clinical and laboratory history, including previous blood gas data if available, can the actual cause be determined.

After treatment for congestive heart failure, his baseline arterial blood gas values reflect a state of chronic respiratory acidosis plus a mild metabolic alkalosis. In retrospect, his blood gas values on admission were the result of acute hyperventilation on top of chronic respiratory acidosis.

8.5. d. A patient can have both vomiting (causing metabolic alkalosis) and uremia (causing metabolic acidosis) at the same time. This patient has renal failure (BUN = 121 mg/dL); the diagnosis of metabolic acidosis is confirmed by the elevated anion gap (25 mEq/L). Despite the AG acidosis, serum CO_2 is elevated at 40 mEq/L (the bicarbonate gap = 26 mEq/L), indicating metabolic alkalosis. In this patient, alkalosis is the dominant condition, hence the blood is alkalemic (pH—7.51). From the information provided, one cannot rule out a primary respiratory acidosis as an additional problem. (After this patient recovered, he showed no evidence of underlying lung disease. Sometimes, it requires days or weeks of follow up to fully characterize acid–base disorders.)

8.6. This patient's blood gas values suggest a state of chronic respiratory alkalosis: very low $PaCO_2$ and slightly elevated pH. This assessment, however, does not indicate a specific diagnosis but only suggests possibilities. Accurate diagnosis must be made in conjunction with the clinical picture plus other laboratory studies. Could this patient have a mixed problem: respiratory alkalosis plus metabolic acidosis? Her anion gap is

$$Na^+ - (Cl^- + CO_2) = 142 - 118 = 24 \text{ mEq/L}$$

The anion gap is elevated and indicates a metabolic acidosis. The acid–base disorder, however, is not *just* metabolic acidosis, because the blood is alkalemic. There is good evidence she has *both* metabolic acidosis *and* respiratory alkalosis, the latter disorder from excessive mechanical ventilation. The cause of metabolic acidosis must be looked for, because it is not apparent from the information provided. Because the anion gap is elevated, the possibilities include lactic acidosis from hypoperfusion and drug-induced metabolic acidosis.

8.7. The patient initially had chronic respiratory alkalosis, resulting from several days of hyperventilation, during which time her kidneys had a chance to excrete bicarbonate and return the pH toward normal. Now her asthmatic condition has worsened; she has acutely hypoventilated. The second set of blood gas values reflects acute respiratory acidosis *on top of* a chronic respiratory alkalosis. Although her bicarbonate is low, there is no primary metabolic process; and treatment must be aimed at her respiratory disorders.

8.8. This patient has more than respiratory acidosis, because the initial calculated bicarbonate is low (21 mEq/L). There is a concomitant metabolic acidosis, confirmed by an elevated anion gap. He has two causes of metabolic acidosis: shock and severe hypoxemia. After intubation, he is ventilated down to a "normal" $PaCO_2$ of 40 mm Hg, a de facto respiratory alkalosis; yet he remains acidemic, because his metabolic process (lactic acidosis) has not been corrected. The last set of blood gas values still shows metabolic acidosis and inadequate respiratory compensation, or what some people would call respiratory acidosis. Note: **The terms *respiratory alkalosis,* for his change in $PaCO_2$ from 70 to 40 mm Hg, and *respiratory acidosis,* for his $PaCO_2$ at 40 mm Hg with metabolic acidosis, are technically correct.**

As long as you understand the changes and how they came about, it is not important how they are labeled; you could just as well use *hyperventilation* instead of respiratory alkalosis and *inadequate respiratory compensation* instead of respiratory acidosis.

8.9.

a. False
b. True
c. True
d. True
e. False
f. True
g. False
h. False

CHAPTER

Putting It All Together

Cases

You are now ready to interpret arterial blood gases in almost any clinical situation. In this chapter are five actual cases managed with the aid of arterial blood gas data. Each case is accompanied by multiple choice questions. For each question, select the *one best answer* (answers with explanations are at the end of the chapter). Remember to use *all available information* in answering each question. For each case, I recommend you answer all the questions first, then check the answers.

MR. A: A CASE OF ACUTE RESPIRATORY DISTRESS *Mr. A is a 25-year-old man who comes to the emergency room complaining of increasing shortness of breath. He has had upper respiratory symptoms—mainly cough, fever, and progressive dyspnea—for three days. On examination, he appears cyanotic and in respiratory distress; inspiratory rales are heard over the left lung base, and his respiratory rate is 40/min. A chest x-ray confirms left lower lobe pneumonia. His temperature is 102°F and white blood cell count 17,000/mm³. Arterial blood gas and serum electrolytes show*

$FIO_2 = 0.21$	$COHb = 1.5\%$
$pH = 7.55$	$Hb = 14$ g/dL
$PaCO_2 = 25$ mm Hg	$Na^+ = 140$ mEq/L
$PaO_2 = 38$ mm Hg	$K^+ = 4.2$ mEq/L
$SaO_2 = 78\%$	$Cl^- = 106$ mEq/L
$HCO_3^- = 21$ mEq/L	$CO_2 = 20$ mEq/L

1. The patient is severely hypoxemic as a result of
   a. hypoventilation and venous admixture
   b. Hyperventilation causing a left shift of the oxygen dissociation curve and reduced SaO_2
   c. Increased methemoglobin

d. Ventilation–perfusion imbalance
e. Decreased cardiac output and oxygen transport

2. Arterial oxygen content, in mL O_2/dL, is approximately
   a. 10
   b. 12.5
   c. 14.6
   d. 16
   e. 18

3. $P(A\text{–}a)O_2$, in mm Hg, is approximately
   a. 15
   b. 82
   c. 108
   d. 145
   e. 662

4. PaO_2/FIO_2 is
   a. 100
   b. 150
   c. 180
   d. 230
   e. 310

5. The patient's acid–base status is best characterized as
   a. Marked hyperventilation and metabolic acidosis
   b. Respiratory alkalosis and metabolic acidosis
   c. Chronic respiratory alkalosis
   d. Acute respiratory alkalosis
   e. Respiratory alkalosis and metabolic alkalosis

6. At this point, in addition to antibiotics, you would treat the patient with
   a. Intravenous bicarbonate and low supplemental oxygen ($FIO_2 < 0.40$) by face mask or nasal cannula
   b. 28% oxygen by Venturi face mask
   c. A non-rebreather face mask to deliver an oxygen concentration > 60%
   d. A mixture of inhaled carbon dioxide and oxygen to lower pH and raise PaO_2 to > 80 mm Hg
   e. Both oxygen by face mask and a blood transfusion to most effectively raise oxygen content

About 12 h later Mr. A appears no better. By this time he is in the intensive care unit and his FIO_2 has been increased to 90% by face mask. His PaO_2, however, is only 55 mm Hg, and the chest x-ray now shows extensive bilateral pneumonia. Diagnosis: acute respiratory distress syndrome from infectious pneumonia, specific cause to be determined. Because of oxygenation failure, he is given some sedation with the drug midazolam; then intubated and provided mechanical ventilation. Ventilator settings include 100% inspired oxygen, assist-control mode at 14 breaths/min, and tidal volume of 600 mL. His total respiratory rate is 20/min, and he appears comfortable. The peak inspiratory pressure is 40 cm H_2O. Blood gas results after 30 min on these settings are

$FIO_2 = 1.00$
pH = 7.40
$PaCO_2 = 25$ mm Hg
$PaO_2 = 60$ mm Hg

$SaO_2 = 85\%$
$HCO_3^- = 15$ mEq/L
Hb = 13 g/dL

7. Now the most likely cause of hypoxemia is
   a. Hypoventilation
   b. A change in the position of his O_2 dissociation curve
   c. Areas of lung with perfusion but no ventilation
   d. Diffusion barrier caused by the pneumonia
   e. None of the above

8. Arterial oxygen content, in mL O_2/dL blood, is
   a. 12.2
   b. 14.8
   c. 16.4
   d. 17.4
   e. Indeterminate from information provided

9. The $P(A–a)O_2$, in mm Hg, is in the range of
   a. 250–275
   b. 350–375
   c. 400–450
   d. 500–550
   e. > 600

10. The PaO_2/FIO_2 is
    a. 60
    b. 120
    c. 180
    d. 250
    e. 300

11. Mr. A's acid–base status at this point is best characterized as
    a. Chronic metabolic acidosis
    b. Chronic respiratory alkalosis
    c. Respiratory alkalosis plus metabolic acidosis
    d. Metabolic acidosis plus respiratory acidosis
    e. Indeterminate from the information provided

12. The best therapeutic approach at this point is to
    a. Transfuse 1 unit of blood
    b. Add positive end-expiratory pressure to the ventilator circuit
    c. Hyperventilate to shift the O_2 dissociation curve to the left
    d. Hypoventilate to shift the O_2 dissociation curve to the right
    e. Paralyze the patient to provide pressure-controlled ventilation

MR. B: A CASE OF CHRONIC OBSTRUCTIVE PULMONARY DISEASE

Mr. B is a 65-year-old man brought to the emergency department in moderate respiratory distress. He has smoked two packs of cigarettes daily for 45 years and has refused to quit, despite pleading by his family and physician. Pulmonary function tests during past outpatient evaluations showed marked airways obstruction consistent with severe chronic obstructive pulmonary disease (COPD). He was said to be "doing well" until a few days earlier when he developed a cough and dyspnea. At that time, he reduced his smoking to about half a pack a day.

Examination in the emergency department reveals cyanotic fingers and lips, bilateral wheezing, and a few scattered rales in the lung bases. Mr. B's respiratory rate is 30/min, and he is using accessory breathing muscles. His feet and legs are edematous, and there is a slight hand tremor. Though in some respiratory distress, Mr. B is alert and oriented. His chest x-ray shows flattened diaphragms and hyperinflation consistent with COPD and no acute infiltrates. Electrocardiogram shows changes consistent with pulmonary hypertension, but no evidence for coronary ischemia. Pulse oximeter SpO_2 (on room air, FIO_2 = 0.21) is 62%. The first set of arterial blood gases and electrolytes shows

FIO_2 = 0.21
pH = 7.36
$PaCO_2$ = 60 mm Hg
PaO_2 = 35 mm Hg
SaO_2 = 51%
HCO_3^- = 33 mEq/L

Hb = 17 g/dL
Na^+ = 140 mEq/L
K^+ = 4.2 mEq/L
Cl^- = 91 mEq/L
CO_2 = 35 mEq/L

1. The most likely physiologic explanation for his hypoxemia is
   a. Right-to-left shunting alone
   b. V–Q imbalance alone
   c. Hypoventilation and V–Q imbalance
   d. Hypoventilation, V–Q imbalance, and increased carbon monoxide level
   e. Diffusion block and V–Q imbalance.

2. At this point you would prescribe
   a. A respiratory stimulant, such as doxapram, plus bicarbonate therapy, inhaled bronchodilator, and steroids, but no supplemental oxygen
   b. Oxygen by face mask at an FIO_2 of 40% or less
   c. Oxygen by face mask as close to 100% as possible
   d. Intubation and mechanical ventilation with whatever FIO_2, is necessary to raise PaO_2 above 60 mm Hg
   e. Phlebotomy of 1 unit of blood and a non-rebreather face mask to deliver maximal inspired oxygen

3. Your answer to question 2 is based on knowledge that
   a. Correcting his underlying condition is the most important part of therapy
   b. A small change in PaO_2 in this region of the oxygen dissociation curve can lead to a relatively large change in SaO_2
   c. In this region of the oxygen dissociation curve, a high FIO_2 is needed to improve the SaO_2
   d. Hypoxemia is life-threatening, and a patient's PaO_2 should be improved as quickly as possible
   e. Removing hemoglobin while adding supplemental oxygen will improve global oxygen transport

Mr. B initially does well on your regimen. However, 6 h later he is much less alert; he falls asleep easily and responds only when vigorously stimulated. Repeat arterial blood gases (on supplemental oxygen) show

pH = 7.10	Na^+ = 140 mEq/L
$PaCO_2$ = 80 mm Hg	K^+ = 4.4 mEq/L
PaO_2 = 40 mm Hg	Cl^- = 90 mEq/L
SaO_2 = 64%	CO_2 = 26 mEq/L
HCO_3^- = 24 mEq/L	

You now conclude that Mr. B requires mechanical ventilation because of altered mental status, hypoventilation, hypoxemia, *and* acidemia.

4. Mr. B's acid–base status before intubation is best characterized as
   a. Acute respiratory acidosis on top of chronic respiratory acidosis, plus metabolic alkalosis
   b. Acute respiratory acidosis on top of chronic respiratory acidosis, plus metabolic acidosis
   c. Chronic respiratory acidosis plus metabolic acidosis
   d. Chronic respiratory acidosis plus metabolic alkalosis
   e. Indeterminate from the information provided

Mr. B is an example of a blue bloater, *a term applied to patients with severe chronic bronchitis who are prone to significant hypoxemia (making them blue or cyanotic) and right-sided heart failure (making them bloated or edematous) during exacerbations of their condition. With good medical management such patients can live for many years. Treatment includes judicious supplemental oxygen, bronchodilators, an occasional course of steroids, and smoking cessation. Potentially lethal are upper respiratory infections, pneumonia, pulmonary embolism, and other acute pulmonary insults. Infection was the presumed cause of Mr. B's decompensation.*

Mr. B's ventilator is set to deliver 16 breaths/min and a tidal volume of 700 mL. Blood gas measurements obtained 1 h later, on an FIO_2 of 40%, show

pH = 7.30	SaO_2 = 90%
$PaCO_2$ = 50 mm Hg	HCO_3^- = 24 mEq/L
PaO_2 = 80 mm Hg	Hb = 16.8 g/dL

5. At this point you would
   a. Give 50 mEq/L of bicarbonate intravenously and repeat the blood gas measurements
   b. Increase FIO_2 to 0.60
   c. Increase tidal volume to 900 mL
   d. Increase breathing frequency to 20/min
   e. Not change the ventilator settings

Over the next few days Mr. B is treated with diuretics, steroids, antibiotics, and chest physiotherapy; and he improves clinically. By the third hospital day, his wheezing has cleared, and he is alert and feeling better. He points to his endotracheal tube and indicates through gestures that he wishes it removed. At this point, the ventilator is set to deliver intermittent mandatory ventilation (IMV) at 6 breaths/min and a tidal volume of 700 mL. His own spontaneous respiratory rate is 10 breaths/min for a total respiratory rate of 16/min. While breathing an FIO_2 of 28%, he has the following blood gas values:

pH = 7.56
$PaCO_2$ = 40 mm Hg
PaO_2 = 65 mm Hg
SaO_2 = 94%
HCO_3^- = 35 mEq/L
Hb = 15 g/dL

6. At this point you would
   a. Extubate him but maintain the same FIO_2
   b. Repeat the blood gas in 6h; and if no worse, extubate him, keeping the same FIO_2
   c. Disconnect him from the ventilator without extubation (e.g., using a "blow-by" or "T-piece" at the same FIO_2), so he can breathe spontaneously through the endotracheal tube; repeat the blood gas in a few hours; and if the results are adequate, then extubate
   d. Remove supplemental oxygen but keep the same ventilator settings; and if his PaO_2 remains adequate, extubate
   e. Decrease the number of IMV breaths per minute while keeping the same FIO_2
7. Your answer to question 6 is based on the fact that
   a. There are a number of complications of intubation, and the endotracheal tube should be removed as soon as possible
   b. Blood gas measurements reflect the patient's gas exchange status at a particular time, and the situation may change rapidly; however, if the blood gas results are essentially the same over a period of time the patient is likely to remain stable
   c. If a patient can breathe on his own through an endotracheal tube, he will also be able to breathe without one
   d. The patient will be breathing room air after discharge, so you must ensure that his blood gas measurements are at least adequate on room air before extubation
   e. The goal is to achieve his baseline state in terms of gas exchange and not to extubate when blood gas results are better than he can manage without ventilatory assistance
8. You would like what additional information at this time (choose the one best answer)?
   a. Chest x-ray
   b. P_{50}
   c. Percent carboxyhemoglobin
   d. Serum potassium
   e. Serum calcium

9. What additional treatment might be necessary at this point (choose the one best answer)?
   a. Antibiotics
   b. Blood transfusion
   c. Increasing FIO_2 to 0.40
   d. Potassium chloride
   e. Calcium gluconate

10. Following extubation and after discharge from the hospital, Mr. B does well, although he continues to smoke. When at his clinical best after discharge, the most likely set of arterial blood gas values he would manifest on room air is
    a. $PaO_2 = 80$, $PaCO_2 = 60$, pH = 7.35, $SaO_2 = 90$
    b. $PaO_2 = 58$, $PaCO_2 = 55$, pH = 7.37, $SaO_2 = 86$
    c. $PaO_2 = 90$, $PaCO_2 = 35$, pH = 7.43, $SaO_2 = 90$
    d. $PaO_2 = 38$, $PaCO_2 = 67$, pH = 7.38, $SaO_2 = 80$
    e. $PaO_2 = 72$, $PaCO_2 = 28$, pH = 7.34, $SaO_2 = 93$

MR. C: A CASE OF INTOXICATION *Mr. C. is a 27-year-old man brought to the emergency department (ED) comatose. He was reportedly found unconscious at home by friends. There is a history of cigarette smoking and a questionable history of drug abuse, but no one stayed around the ED to answer any questions. On examination, he is comatose, breathing at 8/min. Vital signs are stable and his heart rate is 105/min. ECG shows sinus tachycardia with no evidence of coronary ischemia. Arterial blood is sent for blood gas analysis ($FIO_2 = 0.21$), and venous blood is sent for electrolytes and toxicology screen. The arterial blood gas data are first to return and show*

pH = 7.34
$PaCO_2 = 42$ mm Hg
$PaO_2 = 82$ mm Hg
$SaO_2 = 93\%$ (calculated)
$HCO_3^- = 22$ mEq/L
Hb = 16 g/dL

1. What specific information should you obtain at this point (choose the one best answer)?
   a. Anion gap
   b. Serum K^+
   c. Co-oximeter-measured SaO_2
   d. P_{50}
   e. Lactate level

2. Your answer to question 1 is based on the fact that
   a. The anion gap can help determine what type of metabolic acidosis is present
   b. Given a metabolic acidosis, it is important to know if hyperkalemia is present, and to what degree
   c. The calculated oxygen saturation could mask a true reduction in SaO_2
   d. The position of the O_2 dissociation curve is an aid to determine if the patient is adequately oxygenated
   e. Lactate level might indicate a poor perfusion state and help diagnose the cause of coma.

Additional laboratory tests are ordered, and the following results are obtained

SaO_2 = 50% (measured) Lactate = 2.0 mmol/L
COHb = 47%

Just as you receive these results, one of the friends returns to report that Mr. C's cat was found dead in the apartment and that the police and fire department were called. Firemen found high levels of carbon monoxide in the apartment, which they attributed to a faulty space heater. You thank the friend for this belated information and inform him that Mr. C is comatose from acute carbon monoxide intoxication.

3. Mr. C's arterial oxygen content, in ml O_2/dL blood, is approximately
   a. 8.0
   b. 10.9
   c. 11.6
   d. 12.8
   e. Indeterminate without more information
4. The position of his oxygen dissociation curve
   a. Inhibits unloading of oxygen at the tissue level
   b. Inhibits uptake of oxygen at the pulmonary capillary level
   c. Is the same as a patient with normal gas exchange whose hemoglobin content is half of Mr. C's
   d. Is not clinically relevant in this case
   e. Cannot be assessed from the information provided
5. Of the following, which one of the treatment options would you prescribe at this point?
   a. Intubate and give 100% oxygen via a ventilator
   b. Intubate and give 60% oxygen via a ventilator

c. Give 90% oxygen by face mask
d. Give 50% oxygen by face mask
e. Give oxygen via nasal cannula at 3 L/min

A monitor ECG now shows some ischemic cardiac changes, confirmed by a 12-lead ECG. You prescribe intravenous nitroglycerin at a rate of 10 μg/min. Also, he is now receiving 100% inspired oxygen. About 1 h later, arterial blood gas analysis reveals

pH = 7.45
$PaCO_2$ = 30 mm Hg
PaO_2 = 525 mm Hg
SaO_2 = 75%
HCO_3^- = 22 mEq/L
COHb = 25%
Hb = 16 g/dL

6. How would you interpret these blood gas data?
   a. Consistent with improvement from CO intoxication
   b. Suggestive of methemoglobinemia
   c. Suggestive of aspiration pneumonia
   d. He has developed a metabolic acidosis
   e. He has developed evidence of oxygen toxicity

7. What therapeutic intervention would be most appropriate at this point?
   a. Continue FIO_2 at 100%
   b. Intravenous methylprednisolone
   c. Intravenous methylene blue
   d. 100 mEq (2 ampules) of intravenous sodium bicarbonate
   e. Oxygen therapy in a hyperbaric chamber

The next day, after appropriate therapeutic intervention, Mr. C is awake and alert; he has been extubated and disconnected from the ventilator. At this point arterial blood gas data, on 3 L/min nasal oxygen, show

pH = 7.42
$PaCO_2$ = 36 mm Hg
PaO_2 = 124 mm Hg
SaO_2 = 90%
HCO_3^- = 24 mEq/L
COHb = 8%
Hb = 15.8 g/dL

8. His alveolar–arterial PO_2 difference is
   a. Increased
   b. Decreased
   c. Indeterminate from information provided
   d. Not relevant in presence of excess CO
   e. Both c and d

Mr. C is discharged 3 days later, in good physical condition. On a return visit, 2 weeks after discharge, he is asymptomatic. The following blood gases are obtained while he is breathing room air:

pH = 7.41
$PaCO_2$ = 37 mm Hg
PaO_2 = 88 mm Hg
SaO_2 = 91%
HCO_3^- = 24 mEq/L
COHb = 7%
Hb = 15 g/dL

9. A pulse oximetry measurement at this point would likely be
   a. Significantly higher than 91%
   b. Close to 91% (± 1–2%)
   c. Significantly lower than 91%
   d. Dependent on the amount of methemoglobin also present
10. What is the most likely reason for the slightly elevated CO level at this point?
    a. He is still exposed to the faulty space heater
    b. He is still smoking cigarettes
    c. He has developed some diffusion block from the acute insult 2 weeks earlier
    d. He has developed a ventilation–perfusion imbalance from the acute insult 2 weeks earlier
    e. The level is consistent with natural occurrence of CO in the body

MRS. D: A CASE OF VOMITING AND DEHYDRATION *Mrs. D is a 45-year-old alcoholic with several previous hospital admissions for pancreatitis and alcoholic withdrawal symptoms. She presents to the emergency department with a several days' history of vomiting and not eating. On examination she is alert but is dehydrated and hypotensive and complaining of mild abdominal pain. Her chest x-ray shows clear lung fields. Initial arterial blood gas (obtained on room air) and serum chemistry values are as follows:*

pH = 7.47
$PaCO_2$ = 48 mm Hg
PaO_2 = 78 mm Hg
SaO_2 = 92%
HCO_3^- = 34 mEq/L
COHb = 2%
Hb = 10 g/dL
Na^+ = 130 mEq/L
K^+ = 2.9 mEq/L
Cl^- = 77 mEq/L
CO_2 = 33 mEq/L
BUN = 69 mg/dL
Creatinine = 2.6 mg/dL

1. Mrs. D's acid–base status is *best* characterized as
   a. Metabolic alkalosis alone
   b. Metabolic acidosis alone
   c. Metabolic alkalosis *and* metabolic acidosis
   d. Metabolic alkalosis and compensated respiratory acidosis
   e. Compensated respiratory acidosis and metabolic acidosis

She is treated with intravenous normal saline, potassium chloride, and nasogastric (NG) suction. At 6 h later, her arterial blood gas ($FIO_2 = 0.21$), BUN, and electrolyte data show

pH = 7.51	Na^+ = 135 mEq/L
$PaCO_2$ = 43 mm Hg	K^+ = 3.2 mEq/L
PaO_2 = 69 mm Hg	Cl^- = 84 mEq/L
SaO_2 = 91%	CO_2 = 33 mEq/L
HCO_3^- = 33 mEq/L	BUN = 58 mg/dL

2. All of the following have occurred in the interim, *except*
   a. Alkalosis has persisted, in part owing to NG suction
   b. Acidosis has improved owing to saline infusion
   c. The alveolar–arterial PO_2 difference has increased
   d. The anion gap has increased
   e. The oxygen dissociation curve has shifted to the left

The NG tube is removed, and she is given a single 500-mg dose of intravenous acetazolamide. Saline infusion is continued and supplemental oxygen is given by face mask ($FIO_2 = 31\%$). At 12 h later, the following arterial blood gas, BUN, and electrolyte data are obtained.

pH = 7.48	Na^+ = 137 mEq/L
$PaCO_2$ = 39 mm Hg	K^+ = 3.4 mEq/L
PaO_2 = 95 mm Hg	Cl^- = 88 mEq/L
SaO_2 = 96%	CO_2 = 29 mEq/L
HCO_3^- = 28 mEq/L	BUN = 47 mg/dL

3. The dose of acetazolamide has apparently
   a. Improved oxygenation without elevating $PaCO_2$
   b. Increased her serum sodium
   c. Caused a slight metabolic acidosis
   d. Lowered her anion gap
   e. None of the above

By the next day, Mrs. D is considerably better than when admitted. Her blood pressure is normal, and the abdominal pain has ceased. She is no longer receiving supplemental oxygen. Arterial blood gases, BUN, and electrolyte data now show

$pH = 7.45$
$PaCO_2 = 39$ mm Hg
$PaO_2 = 79$ mm Hg
$SaO_2 = 92\%$
$HCO_3^- = 27$ mEq/L

$Na^+ = 139$ mEq/L
$K^+ = 3.9$ mEq/L
$Cl^- = 94$ mEq/L
$CO_2 = 28$ mEq/L
BUN = 37 mg/dL

4. Her acid–base status at this point is best characterized as
   a. Normal
   b. Mild persistent metabolic acidosis and metabolic alkalosis
   c. Mild persistent metabolic acidosis alone
   d. Mild respiratory alkalosis and metabolic alkalosis
   e. Indeterminate without further information

Mrs. D continues to improve and is discharged 4 days later. Serum electrolytes and BUN on the day of discharge show

$Na^+ = 137$ mEq/L
$K^+ = 4.2$ mEq/L
$Cl^- = 100$ mEq/L

$CO_2 = 20$ mEq/L
BUN = 20 mg/dL

5. The BUN and electrolyte data suggest
   a. Normal organ function
   b. Persistent metabolic alkalosis
   c. Persistent metabolic acidosis
   d. A mild respiratory alkalosis
   e. A mild respiratory acidosis

MR. E: A CASE OF PROLONGED VENTILATOR WEANING *Mr. E, a 65-year-old man, has been hospitalized 2 weeks for exacerbation of COPD and pneumonia. He was intubated on the day of admission and has since received continuous mechanical ventilation. Although he has clinically improved, attempts to wean him from the ventilator have been unsuccessful. He underwent a tracheostomy on hospital day 14. Now his physicians wish to discontinue the indwelling arterial line and to manage his blood gases noninvasively.*

An oximeter monitors SaO_2 (SpO_2), and an infrared capnograph is connected to *the ventilator circuit to measure end-tidal PCO_2 ($PetCO_2$). Serial blood gases on day 15 are correlated with SpO_2 and $PetCO_2$ data and show the following*

Range of arterial blood gas data on day 15

FIO_2 = 0.40	HCO_3^- = 32–36 mEq/L
pH = 7.41–7.45	COHb = 1.5–1.8%
$PaCO_2$ = 56–63 mm Hg	MetHb = 0.8–1.0
PaO_2 = 70– 88 mm Hg	Hb = 13.2–13.4 g/dL
SaO_2 = 90–93%	

Range of SpO_2 and $PetCO_2$ data on day 15

$PetCO_2$ = 35–40 mm Hg	SpO_2 = 89–92%

1. The most likely reason for the large difference between $PaCO_2$ and $PetCO_2$ is
   a. An intermittent leak in the ventilator circuit
   b. Dilution of $PetCO_2$ by the high FIO_2
   c. The patient's lung disease
   d. The normal spread between the two values
   e. A faulty capnograph

The arterial line is removed and noninvasive measurements are continued without any ventilator changes. On day 16, Mr. E remains clinically stable, and noninvasive data show:

$PetCO_2$ = 34 mm Hg	SpO_2 = 93%

2. All of the following are now likely correct, *except*
   a. He has adequate oxygen content
   b. He is hyperventilating
   c. He still has a respiratory acidosis
   d. There is an increased $P(A\text{–}a)O_2$
   e. He does not have significant methemoglobinemia

On the afternoon of day 17, the pulse oximeter shows a decline in SpO_2 from 93 to 88% over 1 h. The reduction is confirmed with another pulse oximeter. At the same time, Mr. E's $PetCO_2$ is steady at 38 mm Hg.

3. All of the following could explain the decline in SpO_2 *except*
   a. Increased V–Q imbalance
   b. Reduction in PaO_2

c. Excess carboxyhemoglobin
d. Right shift of the O_2 dissociation curve

Arterial blood and noninvasive measurements obtained on day 17 show

$FIO_2 = 0.40$	COHb = 1.5%
pH = 7.44	MetHb = 7.8%
$PaCO_2 = 60$ mm Hg	Hb = 13.4 g/dL
$PaO_2 = 92$ mm Hg	$PetCO_2 = 38$ mm Hg
$SaO_2 = 86\%$	$SpO_2 = 88\%$
$HCO_3^- = 36$ mEq/L	

4. The very next step should be to
   a. Increase FIO_2
   b. Transfuse the patient
   c. Review all medications carefully
   d. Begin a reducing agent
   e. Change the ventilator settings

After making appropriate adjustments, Mr. E's SpO_2 improves. On day 18, his noninvasive measurements and serum CO_2 show

$PetCO_2 = 36$ mm Hg	Serum $CO_2 = 33$ mEq/L
$SpO_2 = 92\%$	

5. Based on the observed difference between $PaCO_2$ and $PetCO_2$ over the previous 2 days, Mr. E's arterial pH at this point is approximately
   a. 7.32
   b. 7.37
   c. 7.42
   d. 7.49

These values remain steady over the next several days while ventilator settings are adjusted to slowly wean him from the ventilator. At 3 weeks into hospitalization, he is receiving only minimal ventilator support (4 ventilator breaths/min in the IMV mode) and is comfortable. Noninvasive measurements and serum CO_2 show

$FIO_2 = 0.30$	$SpO_2 = 93\%$
$PetCO_2 = 34$ mm Hg	Serum $CO_2 = 36$ mEq/L

6. At this point you wish to let Mr. E breathe spontaneously, i.e., remove the minimal ventilator support while he remains intubated and connected to

the machine only for backup alarms. Your goal is to extubate him if he can safely oxygenate and ventilate without ventilator support. Which of the following is the best method by which to accomplish this goal?

a. Insert an arterial line before removing ventilator support; check blood gas values after 1 h of spontaneous breathing; if they are acceptable, extubate him
b. Do a single-puncture arterial blood gas after 1 h of spontaneous breathing; if the values are acceptable, extubate him
c. Let him breathe spontaneously for 15 min the first hour, then 30 min the next hour, then 45 min the third hour, and then for a full hour; if his noninvasive measurements remain acceptable during each trial, extubate him.
d. Follow the noninvasive measurements and respiratory rate while he is breathing spontaneously; if he remains comfortable and the SpO_2 and $PetCO_2$ are acceptable after about 1 h, extubate him.

ANSWERS TO THE CASE QUESTIONS

Mr. A

1. d. The most common cause of hypoxemia is a V–Q imbalance: abnormal distribution of ventilation to perfusion among the millions of alveolar–capillary units. Answer a is incorrect because the patient is not hypoventilating. Answer b is incorrect because a left-shifted oxygen dissociation curve would give a *higher* SaO_2 at this PaO_2 and, in any case, would not explain the low PaO_2. Answer c is incorrect because there is no reason to suspect methemoglobinemia (SaO_2 is appropriate for this pH and PaO_2). Finally, there is no evidence to support answer e.

2. c.

$$\begin{aligned} CaO_2 &= SaO_2 \times \text{Hb (g/dL)} \times 1.34 \text{ mL } O_2/\text{g Hb} \\ &= 0.78 \times 14 \times 1.34 \\ &= 14.63 \text{ mL } O_2/\text{dL blood} \end{aligned}$$

Since the PaO_2 is only 38 mm Hg, the dissolved fraction can be ignored.

3. b.

$$\begin{aligned} P(A\text{–}a)O_2 &= PAO_2 - PaO_2 \\ PAO_2 &= FIO_2(P_B - 47 \text{ mm Hg}) - 1.2(PaCO_2) \\ &= 0.21(760 - 47) - 1.2(25) = 120 \text{ mm Hg} \\ PaO_2 &= 38 \text{ mm Hg} \end{aligned}$$

Hence

$$P(A–a)O_2 = 120 - 38 = 82 \text{ mm Hg}$$

4. c.

$$PaO_2/FIO_2 = 38/0.21 = 180.95$$

5. d. The low $PaCO_2$ indicates hyperventilation. The slightly low bicarbonate value is consistent with acute hyperventilation. The anion gap of 14 mEq/L is within normal limits. As there is no evidence for metabolic acidosis, answers a and b are incorrect. Answer c is incorrect because a chronic state would give a lower pH and bicarbonate value. Answer e is incorrect because there is no evidence for metabolic alkalosis.

6. c. There is no reason for low supplemental FIO_2, because the patient is not retaining CO_2. Hence answers a, b, and e are inappropriate. Furthermore, transfusion is not indicated since the patient is not anemic. Answer d is incorrect because this mixture will raise the $PaCO_2$, increase the work of breathing, and do nothing to treat the underlying pneumonia.

7. c. The patient has a right-to-left shunt, i.e., some blood is flowing through his lungs that is not being oxygenated. Answer a is incorrect because he is not hypoventilating. Answer b is incorrect because changes in the oxygen dissociation curve would not affect the PaO_2. Answer d is incorrect since 100% oxygen should overcome a diffusion barrier. Finally, answer e is incorrect because shunting *is* evident from the information given. A normal subject breathing 100% oxygen, without significant right-to-left shunting, should have a PaO_2 > 500 mm Hg.

8. b.

$$\begin{aligned} O_2 \text{ content} &= SaO_2 \times Hb \times 1.34 \\ &= 0.85 \times 13 \times 1.34 \\ &= 14.81 \text{ mL } O_2/\text{dL blood} \end{aligned}$$

Since PaO_2 is low (60 mm Hg), the contribution from dissolved oxygen can be ignored.

9. e. While breathing 100% oxygen,

$$\begin{aligned} PAO_2 &= FIO_2\,(P_B - 47) - PaCO_2 \\ &= 1.0\,(713) - 25 = 688 \text{ mm Hg} \\ P(A–a)O_2 &= 688 - 60 = 628 \text{ mm Hg} \end{aligned}$$

Note that the factor 1.2 in the abbreviated alveolar gas equation becomes 1.00 when breathing 100% oxygen, because nitrogen is fully removed from the lungs (see Chapter 4).

10. a.

$$PaO_2/FIO_2 = 60/1.00 = 60$$

11. c. Neither acid–base disorder alone (respiratory alkalosis, metabolic acidosis) would give a pH of 7.40. When combined in the same patient, the two disorders can mask their respective pH changes (low for acidosis, high for alkalosis) and result in a normal pH. Note that the patient is hyperventilating more than expected for this degree of metabolic acidosis and thus has a primary respiratory alkalosis, caused by hypoxemia, pneumonia, and the artificial ventilation.

12. b. There is no compelling reason to transfuse this patient since his hemoglobin content is near normal. As to answers c and d, the patient has a normal pH and any shift of the curve by altering pH can have an unpredictable and adverse effect on the patient. Paralysis is sometimes used in patients who cannot be adequately ventilated, but his $PaCO_2$ is already low. The best answer of the choices given is to add positive end-expiratory pressure (PEEP), a technique that allows better oxygen transfer at the same FIO_2.

Mr. B

1. d. The patient is hypoventilating ($PaCO_2$ is 60 mm Hg), providing at least one reason for the reduced PaO_2. Assuming barometric pressure of 760 mm Hg, $P(A\text{–}a)O_2$ is 43 mm Hg; this is an elevated value breathing room air and indicates ventilation–perfusion imbalance, consistent with COPD.

Note that the pulse oximetry SpO_2 is 62%, whereas the co-oximeter-measured SaO_2 is 51%. This information provides two clues to excess blood carboxyhemoglobin. First, a PaO_2 of 35 mm Hg should give an $SaO_2 > 60\%$ (at pH = 7.36), not 51%. The lower-than-expected SaO_2 indicates that something else must be binding to hemoglobin besides oxygen. In a smoker, excess carbon monoxide is the most likely explanation. Second, the pulse oximeter reads carboxyhemoglobin as oxyhemoglobin; when they are discrepant, as in this case ($SpO_2 > SaO_2$), elevated COHb is strongly suggested. (His COHb was 7.2%.)

Because of the low SaO_2, Mr. B's arterial oxygen content is reduced to about 11.8 mL O_2/dL. He is thus hypoxemic for three reasons: hypoventilation, ventilation–perfusion imbalance, and excess blood carbon monoxide.

2. b. This patient is a CO_2 retainer and hypoxemic, both conditions arising from a severe ventilation–perfusion imbalance. A high FIO_2 can worsen V–Q relationships and cause further increases in $PaCO_2$. (This effect is sometimes called *blunting the hypoxic drive*, but the worsening V–Q imbalance is probably the mechanism because most CO_2-retaining patients given oxygen don't decrease their tidal volume or respiratory rate.) Irrespective of the FIO_2, however, the increase in $PaCO_2$ is usually modest and not a clinically significant problem if the patient is closely observed. The fact is, most patients of this type don't need more than 40% oxygen to improve SaO_2 to a safe level.

3. b. The patient's PaO_2 is on the so-called steep part of the oxygen dissociation curve. Hence a small increment in the PaO_2 will lead to a relatively large increment in SaO_2 (when compared with the flat part of the curve). As a result, oxygen content can increase without worrying about increasing $PaCO_2$ from too high an FIO_2.

4. b. There is plenty of information by which to answer this question. First, his $PaCO_2$ went from 60 to 80 mm Hg in only 6 h, indicating acute respiratory acidosis on top of chronic respiratory acidosis. If his only acid–base problem were acute respiratory acidosis, HCO_3^- should be higher than 24 mEq/L and pH would be about 7.15, not 7.10. Because both pH and HCO_3^- are lower than predicted for acute respiratory acidosis, he must have another acid–base disorder, i.e., metabolic acidosis.

Second, note that serum CO_2 fell from 33 to 24 mEq/L; this documented decrease alone indicates an acute metabolic acidosis (especially when $PaCO_2$ is rising). Third, note the large anion gap, 24 mEq/L, confirming development (since admission) of anion gap acidosis. In this setting, the cause is most likely lactic acidosis. Finally, his bicarbonate gap ($\Delta AG - \Delta CO_2$) is increased at +11 mEq/L, consistent with chronic respiratory acidosis and/or metabolic alkalosis. Chronic respiratory acidosis explains this finding in his case, although there may also be an element of metabolic alkalosis.

5. e. After 1 h of mechanical ventilation, the patient's $PaCO_2$ has decreased from 80 to 50 mm Hg. The patient is in a transient situation and has not reached a steady state in terms of ventilation. Another hour may show further reduction of his $PaCO_2$. Thus it is best to leave the ventilator settings alone and especially to do nothing that will lower the $PaCO_2$ any faster (as may occur from the steps in answers c and d). The step in answer a is unnecessary because the pH is increasing from reduction of $PaCO_2$; extra HCO_3^- may actually cause an unwanted alkalosis as $PaCO_2$ decreases further.

The step in answer b is unwarranted for two reasons: his PaO_2 is adequate while breathing 40% inspired oxygen, and SaO_2 will increase as his pH increases (O_2 dissociation curve shifts to left).

6. e. See the answer to question 7 for Mr. B's case.

7. e. Your goal should be to return the patient's acid–base and ventilatory status close to what it will be while breathing room air, off the ventilator. He now has a metabolic alkalosis, caused by the diuretics and steroids and manifested by high pH and normal $PaCO_2$ (with resulting high HCO_3^-). The compensation for metabolic alkalosis is hypoventilation; if the patient is extubated, or just disconnected from the ventilator and placed on a T-piece, hypoventilation may occur rapidly to compensate the alkalosis. With extubation or a T-piece, the patient may also hypoventilate because of underlying chronic lung disease. We know from his history and presenting arterial blood gas values that he is most likely a chronic carbon dioxide retainer.

One danger of sudden hypoventilation is the rapid fall that can occur in PaO_2 as $PaCO_2$ increases. Optimally one should (1) allow the patient to achieve his baseline state of hypoventilation while being mechanically ventilated so he does not acutely hypoventilate once extubated and (2) remove any metabolic cause of further hypoventilation by aggressively treating the metabolic alkalosis. A safe approach is to decrease the number of IMV breaths/min while correcting the alkalosis. In this way, the patient can gradually hypoventilate while acid–base and oxygen status are closely monitored. Another 24 h of such management might ensure a more successful extubation.

There are many approaches to weaning such patients from the ventilator; of the answers provided here, e seems best for the reasons given above. However, other physicians might opt for answer c, using short T-piece periods to let the patient adjust to being disconnected from the ventilator. However, a few hours may be too long to wait before repeating the blood gas. In managing such cases, it is more important to be aware of the physiologic principles involved and of the clinical response to treatment than to follow rigid rules.

8. d. Because the patient has metabolic alkalosis, you want to evaluate his serum K^+; none of the other tests seem particularly indicated at this time.

9. d. Most likely the patient is hypokalemic because of the diuretic therapy.

10. b. Answer a is incorrect because the patient would not have a PaO_2 of 80 mm Hg with a $PaCO_2$ of 60 mm Hg; such values would constitute a negative $P(A–a)O_2$. Answer c is unlikely since we know he is a chronic CO_2 retainer;

these blood gas measurements show a slightly reduced $PaCO_2$ and a normal PaO_2, values unlikely in a patient with such severe respiratory disease. Answer d is unlikely because the PaO_2 is too low for him to be doing well. On a physiologic basis, this PaO_2 would give an $SaO_2 < 75\%$, not one of 80%. Answer e is unlikely because these blood gas values suggest a metabolic acidosis, which he has no reason to have. Also, it is unlikely he could hyperventilate to this degree and considered to be doing well.

Mr. C

1. c. The calculated SaO_2 may be inaccurate if the position of the oxygen dissociation curve is shifted from normal. The P_{50} would give you this information, but it is a much more complex test to run than is the SaO_2. The other information could be useful but SaO_2 measurement should be obtained first in this case.

2. c. See the answer to question 1 for Mr. C's case.

3. b.

$$\begin{aligned} CaO_2 &= (SaO_2 \times Hb \times 1.34) + (0.003 \times 82) \\ &= (0.50 \times 16 \times 1.34) + 0.25 \\ &= 10.97 \text{ mL } O_2/\text{dL} \end{aligned}$$

Note that the answer is b with or without calculation of the dissolved oxygen fraction.

4. a. His oxygen dissociation curve is shifted to the left, and thus unloading of oxygen is retarded at the tissue level.

5. a. This patient is comatose and critically hypoxemic. Of the options listed, the best is to intubate him and give 100% oxygen via ventilator. A hyperbaric chamber would also be appropriate, but such a device is available in only a minority of hospitals.

6. a. These results are entirely consistent with improvement from CO intoxication; his SaO_2 remains low but is rising as CO is removed from the blood. Because the patient is receiving nitroglycerin, he is at some risk for developing methemoglobinemia. However, the SaO_2 + %COHb total 100%, so there is no evidence for methemoglobin. His PaO_2 is appropriate for someone receiving 100% oxygen, so there is also no reason to suspect aspiration pneumonia. His blood gases do not suggest a metabolic acidosis. Finally, it is too soon to develop oxygen toxicity.

7. a or e. There is no indication for the other three maneuvers. You want to keep the FIO_2 high to eliminate carbon monoxide quickly, and it is too soon to worry about oxygen toxicity. Facilities with a hyperbaric chamber would probably opt for that treatment, because some studies suggest better long-term results when carbon monoxide poisoning is treated with hyperbaric oxygen. However, hyperbaric chambers are not available in most hospitals.

8. c. Nasal oxygen at "3 L/min" is an indeterminate FIO_2, so one cannot calculate the alveolar–arterial PO_2 difference. If the PaO_2 was lower than expected for room air, then answer b would obviously be correct. As for answer e, the alveolar–arterial PO_2 difference is definitely relevant, because an increase could be the first clue to co-existing lung disease or a pulmonary complication (such as aspiration pneumonia).

9. a. Pulse oximetry would read the 7% COHb and the 91% SaO_2 as one value, SpO_2, which would be 98%. Answer d is not correct because with 7% COHb and 91% SaO_2, %MetHb can be no more than 2%.

10. b. Mr. C became comatose from a very high CO level. The level is now only 7%, slightly elevated and consistent with continued cigarette smoking. Neither diffusion block nor V–Q imbalance would cause an elevation of CO; the CO level from natural breakdown of heme is $< 3\%$.

Mrs. D

1. c. The elevated CO_2 and pH indicate a metabolic alkalosis. The anion gap, however, is $130 - (77 + 33) = 20$ mEq/L, giving an excess anion gap (ΔAG) of $20 - 12 = 8$ mEq/L and indicating an anion gap metabolic acidosis as well. In this patient alkalosis is predominating over acidosis, hence the elevated pH.

The anion gap acidosis can be attributed to dehydration, poor tissue perfusion, and perhaps some mild renal insufficiency, although the elevated BUN and creatinine could all be from dehydration. Her metabolic alkalosis can be attributed to vomiting, vascular contraction, and hypokalemia. Finally, the hypercapnia could be solely a compensation for metabolic alkalosis.

2. d. Her anion gap has decreased with volume infusion to $135 - (84 + 33) = 18$ mEq/L. At the same time, metabolic alkalosis has persisted (CO_2 remains elevated at 33 mEq/L), the A–a PO_2 difference has increased, and (because of the higher pH) her O_2 dissociation curve has shifted to the left.

3. c. Acetazolamide is a carbonic anhydrase inhibitor that acidifies the blood by preventing renal reabsorption of bicarbonate. The drug has induced a mild metabolic acidosis, as evidenced by the fall in bicarbonate to 28 mEq/L (CO_2 to 29 mEq/L).

4. b. Her anion gap is still elevated at $139 - (94 + 28) = 17$ mEq/L, suggesting a mild persistent metabolic acidosis. The excess anion gap (ΔAG) of 5 mEq/L, however, should give a low serum CO_2, about 22 mEq/L; Because her CO_2 remains elevated at 28 mEq/L there is still a persistent mild metabolic alkalosis.

5. c. Her anion gap is now $137 - (100 + 20) = 17$ mEq/L, suggesting persistent metabolic acidosis ($\Delta AG = 5$ mEq/L), probably from mild renal insufficiency. At the same time, her ΔCO_2 is $27 - 20 = 7$ mEq, for a bicarbonate gap ($\Delta AG - \Delta CO_2$) of $5 - (-7) = -2$ mEq/L; this value is well within the normal range, indicating that her venous CO_2 is appropriately low and that the metabolic alkalosis has corrected.

Mr. E

1. c. The patient has increased dead space from lung disease and for this reason manifests a large difference between $PaCO_2$ and $PetCO_2$. (The normal difference is 0 to a few mm Hg). Answers a and e are also possible, and the capnograph and its connections should be frequently checked. FIO_2 has no direct effect on $PaCO_2$ or end-tidal PCO_2.

2. b. The initial spread between $PaCO_2$ and $PetCO_2$ was 21–23 mm Hg. There is no reason to expect any change in this difference, so the patient's $PaCO_2$ is still high; he is not hyperventilating. The other answers are correct.

3. c. Carboxyhemoglobin is not measured by pulse oximeters but is read as oxyhemoglobin. Thus an elevation in COHb is not reflected in SpO_2. All the other conditions could lead to a true reduction in SaO_2 and SpO_2.

4. c. This patient now has an increased methemoglobin level. He was receiving acetaminophen (Tylenol), a drug sometimes associated with increased methemoglobin. The drug was discontinued. None of the other steps listed is particularly indicated at this time.

5. b. You can use the Henderson–Hasselbalch equation or the acid–base map (Fig. 8.2). Either way, you need HCO_3^- and $PaCO_2$. For the former, use the total CO_2 of 33 mEq/L. For $PaCO_2$, add the $PaCO_2 - PetCO_2$ difference (about 22 mEq/L) to the most recent $PetCO_2$ measurement (36 mEq/L) to obtain an estimated $PaCO_2$ of 58 mm Hg. These values translate into a pH of 7.37.

6. d. There is no compelling reason to resume measurement of arterial blood gases. Respiratory rate is a good monitor of clinical distress and, with SpO_2 and $PetCO_2$, should provide enough information to monitor the patient when he is breathing spontaneously. In the case described, there is no reason to do the stepped procedure outlined in answer c.

CHAPTER

10

Putting It All Together

Free Text Interpretations

In this chapter are 20 brief clinical descriptions along with blood gas data. In some cases, electrolyte data are also provided. You should interpret all the data for each case in terms of *ventilation, oxygenation* and *acid–base status.* Do those calculations appropriate for your interpretations. Assume barometric pressure is 760 mm Hg.

The specific wording of the interpretations is up to you. Adopt the role of a consultant. Assume another student or physician has just presented the data to you and has asked for your formal interpretation. Make sure you **Write down your interpretations before checking the answer section.** There is a natural tendency to make a "mental interpretation" only, but don't succumb. If you don't write down your response, you will be cheating yourself of a valuable learning exercise.

Do 1 or 2 cases, compare your interpretations with those provided at the end of the chapter, then go back and do some more. I recommend that you not try to complete all 20 cases in one sitting.

CASE 1. *A 55-year-old man is evaluated in the pulmonary lab for shortness of breath. His regular medications include a diuretic for hypertension and one aspirin a day. He smokes a pack of cigarettes a day.*

FIO_2 = 0.21	HCO_3^- = 30 mEq/L
pH = 7.53	COHb = 7.8%
$PaCO_2$ = 37 mm Hg	MetHb = 0.8%
PaO_2 = 62 mm Hg	Hb = 14 g/dL
SaO_2 = 87%	CaO_2 = 16.5 mL O_2/dL

Oxygenation: ______________________________

____

Ventilation: ______________________________

____

Acid–base: ______________________________

____

CASE 2. *A 23-year-old woman is seen in the emergency department for difficulty in breathing. Her lung exam and chest x-ray are normal.*

FIO_2 = 0.21
pH = 7.55
$PaCO_2$ = 25 mm Hg
PaO_2 = 112 mm Hg
SaO_2 = 98%
HCO_3^- = 21 mEq/L
COHb = 1.8%

MetHb = 0.6%
Hb = 13 g/dL
CaO_2 = 17.4 mL O_2/dL
Na^+ = 140 mEq/L
K^+ = 4.1 mEq/L
Cl^- = 106 mEq/L
CO_2 = 22 mEq/L

Oxygenation: ______________________________

____

Ventilation: ______________________________

____

Acid–base: ______________________________

____

CASE 3. *A 60-year-old woman is in the coronary care unit for evaluation of chest pain. She is receiving supplemental oxygen by face mask and her chest x-ray shows pulmonary edema.*

FIO_2 = 0.40
pH = 7.22

HCO_3^- = 15 mEq/L
MetHb = 6.2%

$PaCO_2$ = 38 mm Hg
PaO_2 = 76 mm Hg
SaO_2 = 84%
Hb = 10.8 g/dL
CaO_2 = 12.2 mL O_2/dL
COHb = 2.2%

Oxygenation: ______________________________

____

Ventilation: ______________________________

____

Acid–base: ______________________________

____

CASE 4. *A 46-year-old man has been in the hospital 2 days with pneumonia. He was recovering but has just become diaphoretic, dyspneic, and hypotensive.*

FIO_2 = 3 L/min nasal oxygen
pH = 7.40
$PaCO_2$ = 20 mm Hg
PaO_2 = 80 mm Hg
SaO_2 = 95%
HCO_3^- = 12 mEq/L
COHb = 1.0%
MetHb = 0.2%
Hb = 13.3 g/dL
CaO_2 = 17.2 mL O_2/dL

Oxygenation: ______________________________

____

Ventilation: ______________________________

____

Acid–base: ____________________

____

CASE 5. *A 35-year-old man is in the pulmonary lab for evaluation of dyspnea.*

$FIO_2 = 0.21$
pH = 7.43
$PaCO_2 = 37$ mm Hg
$PaO_2 = 92$ mm Hg
$SaO_2 = 96\%$
$HCO_3^- = 24$ mEq/L
COHb = 1.5%
MetHb = 0.6%
Hb = 14.8 g/dL
$CaO_2 = 19.3$ mL O_2/dL

Oxygenation: ____________________

____

Ventilation: ____________________

____

Acid–base: ____________________

____

CASE 6. *A 44-year-old comatose man is brought to the emergency department. His blood pressure and heart rate are normal.*

$FIO_2 = 0.40$
pH = 7.46
$PaCO_2 = 25$ mm Hg
$PaO_2 = 232$ mm Hg
$SaO_2 = 55\%$
$HCO_3^- = 17$ mEq/L
COHb = 43%
MetHb = 1.2%
Hb = 13.7 g/dL
$CaO_2 = 10.8$ mL O_2/dL
$Na^+ = 136$ mEq/L
$K^+ = 3.8$ mEq/L
$Cl^- = 101$ mEq/L
$CO_2 = 15$ mEq/L

Oxygenation: ______________________________

____

Ventilation: ______________________________

____

Acid–base: ______________________________

____

CASE 7. *A 30-year-old woman is being evaluated in the emergency department for chest pain of sudden onset.*

$FIO_2 = 0.21$
$pH = 7.50$
$PaCO_2 = 30$ mm Hg
$PaO_2 = 85$ mm Hg
$SaO_2 = 95\%$

$HCO_3^- = 23$ mEq/L
$MetHb = 0.3\%$
$Hb = 12$ g/dL
$CaO_2 = 15.5$ mL O_2/dL
$COHb = 1.3\%$

Oxygenation: ______________________________

____

Ventilation: ______________________________

____

Acid–base: ______________________________

____

CASE 8. *A 23-year-old woman is brought in a lethargic state to the emergency room. She has a history of diabetes.*

$FIO_2 = 0.21$
pH = 7.02
$PaCO_2 = 12$ mm Hg
$PaO_2 = 115$ mm Hg
$SaO_2 = 93\%$
$HCO_3^- = 3$ mEq/L

$Na^+ = 136$ mEq/L
$K^+ = 3.8$ mEq/L
$Cl^- = 107$ mEq/L
$CO_2 = 5$ mEq/L
Glucose = 675 mg/dL

Oxygenation: ______________________________

____

Ventilation: ______________________________

____

Acid–base: ______________________________

____

CASE 9. *A 39-year-old man is being evaluated in the outpatient department for a nervous condition. He is noticeably anxious and shaking and has a history of alcoholism. He takes several pills but doesn't know their names.*

$FIO_2 = 0.21$
pH = 7.54
$PaCO_2 = 54$ mm Hg
$PaO_2 = 65$ mm Hg
$SaO_2 = 97\%$
$HCO_3^- = 34$ mEq/L
COHb = 1.1%

Hb = 8 g/dL
$CaO_2 = 10.6$ mL O_2/dL
$Na^+ = 130$ mEq/L
$K^+ = 2.8$ mEq/L
$Cl^- = 84$ mEq/L
$CO_2 = 36$ mEq/L

Oxygenation: ______________________________

____

Ventilation: ______________________________

____

Acid–base: ____

____

CASE 10. *A 58-year-old woman is brought to the emergency room after vomiting up bright red blood. She is mildly hypotensive and is breathing 36 times a minute.*

$FIO_2 = 0.21$
$pH = 7.34$
$PaCO_2 = 35$ mm Hg
$PaO_2 = 69$ mm Hg
$SaO_2 = 88\%$
$HCO_3^- = 20$ mEq/L
$COHb = 6.1\%$
$MetHb = 0.4\%$
$Hb = 4$ g/dL
$CaO_2 = 4.92$ mL O_2/dL

Oxygenation: ____

____

Ventilation: ____

____

Acid–base: ____

____

CASE 11. *A 48-year-old man is being evaluated in the emergency department for acute dyspnea.*

$FIO_2 = 0.21$
$pH = 7.19$
$PaCO_2 = 65$ mm Hg
$PaO_2 = 45$ mm Hg
$SaO_2 = 90\%$
$HCO_3^- = 24$ mEq/L
$COHb = 1.1\%$
$MetHb = 0.4$
$Hb = 15.1$ g/dL
$CaO_2 = 18.3$ mL O_2/dL

Oxygenation: ____

____

Ventilation: ______________________________

____

Acid–base: ______________________________

____

CASE 12. *A 65-year-old woman has become suddenly hypotensive 1 day following surgery for a fractured femur.*

$FIO_2 = 0.21$	$HCO_3^- = 23$ mEq/L
pH = 7.47	COHb = 2.1%
$PaCO_2 = 32$ mm Hg	MetHb = 0.5%
$PaO_2 = 57$ mm Hg	Hb = 11.5 g/dL
$SaO_2 = 83\%$	$CaO_2 = 12.9$ mL O_2/dL

Her arterial blood gas before surgery (on room air) showed $PaO_2 = 84$ *mm Hg and* $PaCO_2 = 39$ *mm Hg.*

Oxygenation: ______________________________

____

Ventilation: ______________________________

____

Acid–base: ______________________________

____

CASE 13. *The following arterial blood gas data were obtained during a cardiopulmonary resuscitation.*

$FIO_2 = 1.00$ (via manual bagging)	$HCO_3^- = 20$ mEq/L
pH = 7.10	COHb = 2.1%

$PaCO_2$ = 76 mm Hg
PaO_2 = 125 mm Hg
SaO_2 = 99%
MetHb = 0.5%
Hb = 12 g/dL
CaO_2 = 16.3 mL O_2/dL

Oxygenation: ______________________________

____

Ventilation: ______________________________

____

Acid–base: ______________________________

____

CASE 14. *A 28-year-old woman is in the emergency department following an attempted suicide with aspirin.*

FIO_2 = 0.40
pH = 7.35
$PaCO_2$ = 16 mm Hg
PaO_2 = 130 mm Hg
SaO_2 = 98%
HCO_3^- = 15 mEq/L
COHb = 1.1%
MetHb = 0.5%
Hb = 12.6 g/dL
CaO_2 = 16.9 mL O_2/dL
Na^+ = 140 mEq/L
K^+ = 4.1 mEq/L
Cl^- = 100 mEq/L
CO_2 = 16 mEq/L

Oxygenation: ______________________________

____

Ventilation: ______________________________

____

Acid–base: ______________________________

____

CASE 15. *A 65-year-old man is evaluated for marked obesity and hypertension in the outpatient clinic. His chief complaint is shortness of breath on exertion.*

FIO_2 = 0.21	HCO_3^- = 30 mEq/L
pH = 7.33	COHb = 4.1%
$PaCO_2$ = 59 mm Hg	MetHb = 0.5%
PaO_2 = 54 mm Hg	Hb = 18 g/dL
SaO_2 = 89%	CaO_2 = 21.6 mL O_2/dL

Oxygenation: ______________________________

____

Ventilation: ______________________________

____

Acid–base: ______________________________

____

CASE 16. *Shortly after gastrointestinal endoscopy, a 55-year-old man is noted to increase his respiratory rate and turn blue. Before endoscopy, his room air blood gas was normal.*

FIO_2 = 0.21	HCO_3^- = 16 mEq/L
pH = 7.34	COHb = 1.1%
$PaCO_2$ = 31 mm Hg	MetHb = 18%
PaO_2 = 79 mm Hg	Hb = 11.1 g/dL
SaO_2 = 75%	CaO_2 = 11.4 mL O_2/dL

Oxygenation: ______________________________

____

Ventilation: ______________________________

____

Acid–base: ______________________________

____

CASE 17. *A 70-year-old man is intubated for respiratory failure; the ventilator settings include tidal volume = 700 mL and assist-control mode = 14 breaths/min.*

FIO_2 = 0.40
pH = 7.34
$PaCO_2$ = 48 mm Hg
PaO_2 = 80 mm Hg
SaO_2 = 95%
HCO_3^- = 25 mEq/L
COHb = 2.1%
MetHb = 1.1%
Hb = 14.5 g/dL
CaO_2 = 18.7 mL O_2/dL

Oxygenation: ______________________________

____

Ventilation: ______________________________

____

Acid–base: ______________________________

____

CASE 18. *A 23-year-old man is being evaluated in the emergency room for severe pneumonia. His respiratory rate is 38/min, and he is using accessory breathing muscles.*

FIO_2 = 0.90
pH = 7.29
$PaCO_2$ = 55 mm Hg
PaO_2 = 47 mm Hg
SaO_2 = 86%
HCO_3^- = 23 mEq/L
COHb = 2.1%
MetHb = 1.1%
Hb = 13 g/dL
CaO_2 = 15.8 mL O_2/dL
Na^+ = 154 mEq/L
K^+ = 4.1 mEq/L
Cl^- = 100 mEq/L
CO_2 = 24 mEq/L

Oxygenation: ______________________________

____

Ventilation: ______________________________

____

Acid–base: ______________________________

____

CASE 19. *An arterial blood gas is obtained before and during a treadmill exercise test in a 39-year-old man without any known respiratory problem.*

MEASUREMENT	BEFORE EXERCISE	DURING EXERCISE
Respiratory rate/min	12	30
FIO_2	0.21	0.21
pH	7.43	7.41
$PaCO_2$ (mm Hg)	39	37
PaO_2 (mm Hg)	96	98
SaO_2 (%)	95	95
HCO_3^- (mEq/L)	24	24

Oxygenation: ______________________________

____

Ventilation: ______________________________

____

Acid–base: ______________________________

____

CASE 20. *An arterial blood gas is obtained before and during a treadmill exercise test in a 55-year-old man with severe COPD.*

MEASURE	BEFORE EXERCISE	DURING EXERCISE
Respiratory rate/min	12	40
FIO_2	0.21	0.21
pH	7.38	7.32
$PaCO_2$ (mm Hg)	42	51
PaO_2 (mm Hg)	72	55
SaO_2 (%)	92	83
HCO_3^- (mEq/L)	24	25

Oxygenation: ______________________________

____

Ventilation: ______________________________

____

Acid–base: ______________________________

____

FREE TEXT INTERPRETATIONS

Case 1.

Oxygenation: The PaO_2 and SaO_2 are both reduced on room air. The $P(A–a)O_2$ is elevated (approximately 43 mm Hg), so the low PaO_2 can be attributed to a V–Q imbalance, i.e., a pulmonary problem. The SaO_2 is reduced, in part from the low PaO_2 but mainly from elevated carboxyhemoglobin, which in turn can be attributed to cigarettes. The arterial oxygen content is adequate.

Ventilation: Adequate for the patient's level of CO_2 production; the patient is neither hyperventilating nor hypoventilating.

Acid–base: Elevated pH and HCO_3^- suggest a state of metabolic alkalosis, most likely related to the patient's diuretic; his serum K^+ should be checked for hypokalemia.

Case 2.

Oxygenation: The PaO_2 is normal on room air for this degree of hyperventilation, and her oxygen content is adequate.

Ventilation: She is hyperventilating.

Acid–base: High pH and low $PaCO_2$ are consistent with acute respiratory alkalosis. The slightly low HCO_3^- is expected solely from acute hyperventilation and does not signify a metabolic acidosis. In line with this, her serum electrolytes are normal, and there is no elevation of the anion gap.

Case 3.

Oxygenation: The $P(A–a)O_2$ is elevated on 40% oxygen, consistent with V–Q imbalance from pulmonary edema. The SaO_2 is reduced because of a rightward shift of the oxygen dissociation curve (as a result of acidemia) and an elevated methemoglobin. The elevated methemoglobin may be related to drug therapy. Is she on nitrates? Her oxygen content is reduced from both low SaO_2 and anemia.

Ventilation: The patient has normal alveolar ventilation, which seems clinically inappropriate in view of her apparent metabolic acidosis.

Acid–base: Low pH and normal $PaCO_2$ suggest severe metabolic acidosis with inadequate respiratory compensation; the patient is at risk for developing hypercapnia and respiratory failure.

Case 4.

Oxygenation: The PaO_2 is lower than expected for someone hyperventilating to this degree and receiving supplemental oxygen, and points to a significant V–Q imbalance. The oxygen content is adequate.

Ventilation: $PaCO_2$ is half normal and indicates marked hyperventilation.

Acid–base: Normal pH and very low bicarbonate and $PaCO_2$ indicate a combined respiratory alkalosis and metabolic acidosis. If these changes are of sudden onset, the diagnosis of sepsis should be strongly considered, especially in someone with a documented infection.

Case 5.

Oxygenation: PaO_2 and SaO_2 are within normal limits; there is no evidence for resting hypoxemia.

Ventilation: Within normal limits.

Acid–base: Within normal limits. In summary, these are normal resting arterial blood gases.

Case 6.

Oxygenation: The PaO_2 is increased appropriately for 40% inspired oxygen, suggesting no significant V–Q imbalance. The patient's SaO_2, however, is markedly reduced owing to a carboxyhemoglobin level of 43%. As a result, the oxygen content is reduced. Oxygen delivery in this patient may be markedly compromised because of alkalemia and elevated CO, both factors that shift the oxygen dissociation curve to the left (i.e., cause hemoglobin to hold oxygen more tightly than normal).

Ventilation: The patient is hyperventilating.

Acid–base: Slightly elevated pH with low $PaCO_2$ and low bicarbonate could represent either chronic respiratory alkalosis or respiratory alkalosis plus metabolic acidosis. Because the patient's anion gap is elevated (20 mEq/L), respiratory alkalosis plus metabolic acidosis is more likely.

Case 7.

Oxygenation: The PaO_2 is adequate, but the $P(A\text{–}a)O_2$ is increased (approximately 29 mm Hg), indicating a V–Q imbalance. The symptom of chest pain suggests pulmonary embolism as a possible diagnosis. The oxygen content is adequate.

Ventilation: Hyperventilation.

Acid–base: Consistent with acute respiratory alkalosis.

Case 8.

Oxygenation: The PaO_2 is appropriately increased above normal owing to extreme hyperventilation. The SaO_2 is slightly reduced for this PaO_2 (because of a rightward shift of the oxygen dissociation curve from acidemia) but is nonetheless adequate, as is the patient's oxygen content.

Ventilation: The $PaCO_2$ is very low, indicating extreme hyperventilation; she is at or near the limit of compensation for severe metabolic acidosis.

Acid–base: The pH and $PaCO_2$ are consistent with severe diabetic ketoacidosis. The anion gap is elevated at 24 mEq/L, indicating anion gap acidosis from excess ketoacids, but the ΔAG (12 mEq/L) doesn't fully explain her degree of acidosis (expected CO_2 from ΔAG alone would be at 15 mEq/L). The Bicarbonate gap ($\Delta AG - \Delta CO_2$) is $(12 - 22) = -10$ mEq/L, indicating a coexisting hyperchloremic metabolic acidosis, which could be from kidney disease or diarrhea.

Case 9.

Oxygenation: The PaO_2 is reduced but the SaO_2 is normal, owing to a leftward shift of the oxygen dissociation curve. The patient is markedly anemic; and as a result, his oxygen content is reduced.

Ventilation: The patient is hypoventilating.

Acid–base: Elevated pH and $PaCO_2$ suggest both metabolic alkalosis and respiratory acidosis. Serum electrolytes show both hypokalemia and hyponatremia with a normal anion gap, a situation that could be caused by diuretic use. Hypoventilation could be a compensatory response to metabolic alkalosis.

Case 10.

Oxygenation: The PaO_2 is reduced on room air, indicating a V–Q imbalance. Her SaO_2 is further reduced from an elevated carbon monoxide level. Finally, the oxygen content is markedly reduced, in part owing to the low SaO_2 but mainly because of severe anemia.

Ventilation: The $PaCO_2$ is low normal but may reflect mild hyperventilation owing to metabolic acidosis.

Acid–base: The pH and $PaCO_2$ suggest a mild metabolic acidosis, most likely related to the patient's hypotension and hypoxemia (low oxygen content).

Case 11.

Oxygenation: The patient's PaO_2 is reduced for two reasons: hypercapnia and V-Q imbalance, the latter apparent from an elevated $P(A–a)O_2$ (approximately 27 mm Hg).

Ventilation: The patient is hypoventilating.

Acid–base: The pH and $PaCO_2$ suggest acute respiratory acidosis plus metabolic acidosis; the calculated HCO_3^- is lower than expected from acute respiratory acidosis alone.

Case 12.

Oxygenation: The PaO_2 is very low on room air, owing to a V–Q imbalance. Given her prior normal PaO_2, an acute pulmonary event has occurred. Considering her postoperative status, the most likely diagnosis is acute pulmonary embolism; and a lung scan is clearly indicated. In addition, her oxygen content is slightly reduced, from both low SaO_2 and anemia.

Ventilation: She is hyperventilating.

Acid–base: High pH and low $PaCO_2$ are consistent with acute uncomplicated respiratory alkalosis.

Case 13.

Oxygenation: On 100% oxygen via Ambu bag, the patient has a large $P(A–a)O_2$, indicating significant right-to-left shunting. The oxygen content was adequate at the time the blood gas was obtained.

Ventilation: The patient is not being adequately ventilated by the Ambu bag.

Acid–base: This pH and $PaCO_2$ indicate acute respiratory acidosis plus metabolic acidosis; acute hypoventilation to a $PaCO_2$ of 76 mm Hg alone would lead to a pH > 7.10 and an $HCO_3^- > 20$ mEq/L.

Case 14.

Oxygenation: The PaO_2 is adequate but reduced for this FIO_2, indicating a state of V–Q imbalance. In an overdose situation, one should consider, among other possibilities, aspiration pneumonia. The oxygen content is adequate.

Ventilation: The patient is markedly hyperventilating.

Acid–base: The pH and $PaCO_2$ are consistent with combined respiratory alkalosis and metabolic acidosis, a state often seen in aspirin overdose. The anion gap is elevated at 24 mEq/L, also indicating metabolic acidosis.

Case 15.

Oxygenation: This patient has a low PaO_2 for two reasons: a V–Q imbalance (apparent from the elevated $P(A–a)O_2$) and hypercapnia. His oxygen content is adequate only because of polycythemia, which in turn is most likely related to chronically low PaO_2.

Ventilation: The patient is hypoventilating, perhaps related to obesity.

Acid–base: Consistent with partially compensated respiratory acidosis.

Case 16.

Oxygenation: The patient's PaO_2 is slightly low, but his SaO_2 is much lower than expected for this PaO_2, owing to an elevated methemoglobin level; this in turn is most likely related to a reaction from the local anesthetic used during the procedure (e.g., benzocaine). His oxygen content is low from both low SaO_2 and anemia.

Ventilation: He is hyperventilating.

Acid–base: This patient has developed a mild metabolic acidosis, most likely related to sudden onset of hypoxemia.

Case 17.

Oxygenation: This patient's PaO_2 is adequate but much lower than expected for an FIO_2 of 0.40, indicating a significant V–Q imbalance. His SaO_2 and oxygen content are adequate.

Ventilation: The patient is being slightly hypoventilated by the ventilator.

Acid–base: This pH and $PaCO_2$ suggest mild acute respiratory acidosis. The ventilator settings should be increased to improve alveolar ventilation, lower $PaCO_2$, and increase pH.

Case 18.

Oxygenation: The PaO_2 and SaO_2 are both markedly reduced on 90% inspired oxygen, indicating severe ventilation–perfusion imbalance.

Ventilation: The patient is hypoventilating, despite the presence of tachypnea, indicating significant dead space ventilation. This is a dangerous situation that suggests the need for mechanical ventilation.

Acid–base: The low pH, high $PaCO_2$, and slightly low calculated HCO_3^- all point to combined acute respiratory acidosis and metabolic acidosis. The anion gap is elevated to 30 mEq/L, indicating a clinically significant anion gap acidosis, possibly from lactic acidosis. The bicarbonate gap ($\Delta AG - \Delta CO_2$) is $(18 - 3) = 15$ mEq/L, indicating a significant metabolic alkalosis as well, cause yet undetermined. In summary this patient has respiratory acidosis, metabolic acidosis, and metabolic alkalosis.

Case 19.

Oxygenation: The PaO_2 and SaO_2 are normal both before and during exercise; there is no oxygen desaturation with this level of exercise.

Ventilation: There is normal alveolar ventilation before the treadmill exercise. During exercise, the alveolar ventilation remains adequate for the increase in CO_2 production.

Acid–base: Normal before and during exercise. In summary, this is a normal blood gas response to submaximal exercise; neither the PaO_2 nor the $PaCO_2$ change significantly.

Case 20.

Oxygenation: Before exercise, the PaO_2 and SaO_2 are slightly reduced on room air. During exercise, the PaO_2 falls significantly, possibly reflecting diffusion impairment from the patient's COPD.

Ventilation: There is normal alveolar ventilation before exercise. During exercise, the $PaCO_2$ increases, reflecting inadequate alveolar ventilation for the increase in CO_2 production that accompanies exercise.

Acid–base: Normal before exercise. During exercise, the patient becomes hypercapnic from inadequate alveolar ventilation and develops acute respiratory acidosis.

CHAPTER

11

Putting It All Together

Clinical Evaluation and Test Ordering

The previous two chapters gave you blood gas data to interpret but did not address the more primary question: When is a blood gas indicated? and the related question: Can some other test substitute? Equal in importance to interpreting the data is knowing when—and which—tests of gas exchange should be obtained.

This chapter presents 16 brief cases. For each, you are asked to determine which tests of gas exchange, if any, are indicated. Basically, for each scenario you should decide if there is sufficient concern about the patient's oxygenation, ventilation, and/or acid–base status to obtain an arterial blood gas or some other test. If so, you should specify just what tests are needed, for example:

- Complete arterial blood gas measurements
- Blood gases without co-oximetry
- Co-oximetry alone or some aspect of it
- Pulse oximetry
- End-tidal PCO_2
- Electrolyte measurements
- Some other test(s)

In several of these cases (as in real life) there may be no single best test; more than one test may give the information needed to manage the patient's problem. In some cases, no test (or no additional test) may be needed. **I cannot overemphasize that no matter how comfortable you may feel with any of the scenarios presented here, you should write down your response before checking my answers.** Only in this way will you commit to thinking hard about the question and, as a result, get the most out of the exercise.

CASE 1. *A 45-year-old man comes to the emergency department (ED) complaining of sudden onset of shortness of breath and chest pain. He is ashen in appearance, and his blood pressure is 100/60 mm Hg. Electrocardiogram shows elevated ST segments indicative of myocardial injury.*

How would you assess his oxygenation, ventilation, and acid–base status?

Your response: ______________________________

____

____

____

CASE 2. *A-23-year-old woman comes to the ED complaining of pleuritic chest pain. There is clinical suspicion for pulmonary embolism.*

What, if any, gas exchange measurements should be made?

Your response: ______________________________

____

____

____

CASE 3. *A 65-year-old woman is admitted to the hospital for asthma exacerbation. Two days later she develops some increasing dyspnea, and her peak expiratory flow rate falls. Though alert and oriented, her breathing is uncomfortable, and persistent wheezing is noted on auscultation. Her respiratory rate = 30/min, heart rate = 112/min, and blood pressure = 145/90 mm Hg. Arterial blood gases obtained on nasal oxygen at 3 L/min show*

PaO_2 = 35 mm Hg
SaO_2 = 71% (calculated)

$PaCO_2$ = 54 mm Hg
pH = 7.31

What should be done next?

Your response: ______________________________

____

____

____

CASE 4. *A 27-year-old man is rescued from a store fire and brought to the ED by the emergency squad. He is in no distress but is complaining of headache, and there is some soot on his face. Pulse oximetry SpO_2 is 97%. His vital signs are stable, and he is adamant about wanting to go home and be with his family. His chest x-ray is clear.*

Do any more tests need to be done?

Your response: ______________________________

____

____

____

CASE 5. *An 18-year-old man is brought to the ED after fainting during a church service. He has no past medical history. His sister, who accompanies him, says he started "getting anxious and breathing hard" during gospel singing. The exam reveals a young, healthy-appearing man who is tachypneic and hyperpneic; he has some carpopedal spasm of his fingers. There are no focal neurologic signs, and the cardiopulmonary exam is normal. Pulse oximetry measurement is 99%.*

What, if any, other tests of gas exchange or acid–base balance should be done?

Your response: ______________________________

____

____

____

CASE 6. *A 35-year-old, nonsmoking woman is evaluated in the clinic for asthma. She complains of dyspnea on the slightest exertion. Her peak expiratory flow rate is 60% of predicted. Heart rate = 100/min and respiratory rate = 24/min. Her blood pressure is normal, and she is not using accessory breathing muscles.*

What measurements should be made to assess gas exchange?

Your response: ______________________________

____

____

____

CASE 7. *For 6 days, a 61-year-old man has been in the ICU for respiratory failure, receiving mechanical ventilation. His condition has improved, and he is now being weaned from the ventilator. Shown below are data taken on his 6th hospital day from a single arterial blood gas (10 A.M.) and from several noninvasive measurements (between 10 A.M. and 2 P.M.).*

The 2:00 P.M. measurements were taken while the patient was still connected to the ventilator circuit, but without any IMV breaths (i.e., all breathing was spontaneous). In this mode, he appears comfortable and indicates on a writing pad that he wants the endotracheal tube removed.

	TIME MEASUREMENT WAS TAKEN			
VALUE	10:00 A.M.	Noon	1:00 P.M.	2:00 P.M.
SpO_2 (%)	96	96	95	95
$PetCO_2$ (mm Hg)	30	32	32	31
SpO_2 (%)	96	96	95	95
$PetCO_2$ (mm Hg)	30	32	32	31
FIO_2	0.35	0.35	0.35	0.35
IMV (ventilator breaths/min)	6	6	4	None
Total RR	14	14	12	15
pH	7.45			
$PaCO_2$ (mm Hg)	35			
PaO_2 (mm Hg)	77			
SaO_2 (%)	93			

IMV, intermittent mandatory ventilation; *Total RR,* respiratory rate/minute (includes mechanical ventilator breaths).

Before doing so what additional measurements, if any, should be made?

Your response: ______________________________

____

____

____

CASE 8. *A 62-year-old man is seen in the ED for lethargy and dehydration. Venous blood measurements show the following values:*

$Na^+ = 140$ mEq/L
$K^+ = 4.8$ mEq/L
$Cl^- = 90$ mEq/L
$CO_2 = 24$ mEq/L

$SpO_2 = 95\%$ ($FIO_2 = 0.21$)
BUN = 88 mg/dL
Creatinine = 2.1 mg/dL

Is there any indication for measuring arterial blood gases?

Your response:

CASE 9. *A 23-year-old insulin-dependent diabetic man complaining of fatigue and malaise is seen in the ED. He has skipped his insulin injections the previous 2 days. In the ED, the following venous and arterial blood values are obtained.*

VENOUS BLOOD	ARTERIAL BLOOD (FIO_2 = 0.21)
Blood sugar = 845 mg/dL	pH = 7.10
BUN = 35 mg/dL	$PaCO_2$ = 10 mm Hg
Creatinine = 1.1 mg/dL	PO_2 = 112 mm Hg
Na^+ = 140 mEq/L	HCO_3^- = 4 mEq/L
K^+ = 4.1 mEq/L	
Cl^- = 105 mEq/L	
CO_2 = 5 mEq/L	
Positive for ketones	

The patient is started on intravenous insulin and fluids.

How should one follow his acid–base disorder?

Your response:

CASE 10. *A Fortune 500 company requires one of its executives, a 45-year-old man, to undergo a physical examination before his taking a new position. As part of the exam the company requests "complete pulmonary function tests." He is a lifelong nonsmoker and has no respiratory complaints. Vital capacity and other components of the tests are normal; pulse oximetry* SpO_2 *is 98% on room air.*

Should he also have an arterial blood gas measurement to establish a baseline?

Your response: ______________________________

____

____

____

CASE 11. *A 55-year-old man is being evaluated for a worker's compensation claim for chronic bronchitis. He says he used to smoke heavily but quit 5 years earlier. There is, however, the distinct smell of cigarettes on his clothes. His pulmonary function tests show severe air flow obstruction.*

What tests of gas exchange should be done?

Your response: ______________________________

____

____

____

CASE 12. *A 71-year-old woman is in the ICU for acute pulmonary edema following a heart attack. She is receiving mechanical ventilation (*$FIO_2 = 0.50$*). Other therapy includes intravenous nitroglycerine, digoxin, and furosemide. Gas exchange mon-*

itoring is by both continuous pulse oximetry and capnography; for the past 12 h these measures have been in the range 92–96% for SpO_2 and 30–34 mm Hg for $PetCO_2$.

At 9 A.M. an arterial blood gas showed $PaO_2 = 88$ mm Hg, $PaCO_2 = 34$ mm Hg, and $SaO_2 = 98\%$. At noon, for the first time, her skin and mucous membranes are noted to have a deep bluish tinge. Otherwise, she appears unchanged, with SpO_2 and $PetCO_2$ in the same range as before.

What tests of gas exchange, if any, should be obtained?

Your response: ______________________________

____

____

____

CASE 13. *You are reviewing routine lab data on one of your patients, a 54-year-old woman whose complaint is shortness of breath on climbing stairs. The data show a hemoglobin value of 18 g/dL (normal 12–15 g/dL).*

What additional test(s) should be ordered?

Your response: ______________________________

____

____

____

CASE 14. *A 73-year-old woman is admitted to the hospital with dehydration and urinary tract infection. She is on multiple medications at the nursing home, including drugs for blood pressure, heart disease, glaucoma, and bronchitis. Admission lab values reveal the following electrolytes:*

Na^+ = 156 mEq/L	Cl^- = 100 mEq/L
K^+ = 3.3 mEq/L	CO_2 = 35 mEq/L

What additional tests, if any should be ordered?

Your response: ______________________

____

____

____

CASE 15. *A 45-year-old man is being evaluated in the neurology clinic for chronic headaches. The brain scan and neurologic exam are normal. Among the lab results so far obtained are the following (FIO_2 = .21):*

Pulse oximetry
SpO_2 = 97%

Arterial blood gases

pH = 7.43	HCO_3^- = 24 mEq/L
$PaCO_2$ = 37 mm Hg	FIO_2 = 0.21
PO_2 = 90 mm Hg	

What additional tests, if any, should be ordered?

Your response: ______________________

____

____

____

CASE 16. *A 25-year-old female nurse is being evaluated in the ED for chronic dyspnea. There is a history of vague chest discomfort associated with the dyspnea. Her symptoms have been present about 3 weeks, but she has been able to continue working. She is a nonsmoker and takes no medications. Physical exam, chest x-ray, and electrocardiogram are normal. Pulse oximetry SpO_2 is 98%. Concerned about the possibility of some type of occult lung disease, the physician obtains an arterial blood gas, which shows*

pH = 7.41	HCO_3^- = 23 mEq/L
$PaCO_2$ = 37 mm Hg	FIO_2 = 0.21
PaO_2 = 94 mm Hg	

Although the arterial blood gas shows no defect in gas exchange, the physician remains concerned about the cause of her symptoms and orders a ventilation–perfusion lung scan. This test is normal.

Before reassuring her that everything looks normal, would you order any more tests?

Your response:

___

___

___

ANSWERS

1. You should obtain both a complete arterial blood gas analysis and serum electrolytes, as his clinical state demands quick assessment of oxygenation, ventilation, and acid–base balance. Even before that, however, the patient should already be receiving supplemental oxygen, because of a suspected myocardial infarction (MI). The blood gas should be interpreted in light of the amount of supplemental O_2 being delivered.

2. Complete arterial blood gas is indicated. At the least, you need to determine her $P(A–a)O_2$. An elevated $P(A–a)O_2$ may be a clue to pulmonary embolism, whereas a normal value would argue against (but not completely rule out) the diagnosis. Co-oximetry measurements would indicate any elevation of CO.

3. It is unlikely that her PaO_2 would be 35 mm Hg, given the clinical description and the use of supplemental oxygen; the values are most likely from a venous blood sample. A quick check with pulse oximetry is indicated to confirm that her SaO_2 is higher than the calculated value of 71%. Even if the sample is venous, the pH and $PaCO_2$ should be similar to arterial values, so this patient needs aggressive management of her asthma with monitoring in an intensive care unit.

4. Definitely. He is likely suffering from carbon monoxide intoxication. An arterial blood gas with co-oximetry is mandatory to check for both impairment of pulmonary gas exchange and carbon monoxide levels. Irrespective of the results, this patient should be admitted to the hospital for observation. He is at risk for developing both upper airway inflammation and delayed pulmonary edema.

5. None, as long as he rapidly improves. The clinical description is one of classic anxiety hyperventilation syndrome, which usually responds to treatment with rebreathing from a paper bag, reassurance, and (occasionally) antianxiety medication. He surely has acute respiratory alkalosis. If he doesn't improve with treatment, then a blood gas would be indicated.

6. Pulse oximetry alone should be sufficient to assess gas exchange. As a rule CO_2 retention from asthma doesn't occur at peak flow values $> 50\%$ predicted, and SaO_2 is usually normal or only slightly low during an asthma exacerbation. Because she is a nonsmoker and CO poisoning isn't suspected, the %COHb doesn't have to be checked. Pulse oximetry will be adequate, unless the SpO_2 is unexpectedly very low (e.g., $< 92\%$ on room air), in which case a blood gas should be obtained. Of course, if her asthma worsens during treatment, then a blood gas might also be indicated.

7. The endotracheal tube can be removed without making any additional measurements. The SpO_2 and $PetCO_2$ are stable and, in this case, are reliable surrogates for SaO_2 and $PaCO_2$. Their values and the fact that he breathes on his own without difficulty indicate he no longer needs mechanical ventilation.

8. Yes, arterial blood gases should be measured. Anion gap is 26 mEq/L, indicating a metabolic acidosis. His bicarbonate gap is +11 mEq/L, indicating metabolic alkalosis and/or compensated respiratory acidosis. Unraveling this complex acid–base disorder and properly assessing its severity can be done only by measuring pH and $PaCO_2$.

9. This is an uncomplicated metabolic acidosis from diabetic ketoacidosis (DKA). It is fully compensated in terms of ventilatory response (note that the last two digits of pH = $PaCO_2$). In uncomplicated DKA, it is not necessary to follow arterial blood gases. For purposes of monitoring improvement from acidosis, it is necessary to follow only the venous CO_2 and the anion gap (now 30 mEq/L).

10. An arterial blood gas is not indicated. There is actually no reason in this case to even be concerned about his state of oxygenation. Furthermore, given the normal SpO_2, there is certainly no reason to do an arterial blood gas.

11. A complete blood gas, including co-oximetry, is indicated. The scenario described suggests he is still smoking, and his CO level will be increased.

12. This scenario suggests sudden development of methemoglobinemia, most likely from IV nitroglycerine. Methemoglobin imparts a cyanotic color to the skin. The complete blood gas should now be repeated, including a co-oximetry measurement for %MetHb.

13. This patient's hemoglobin is elevated, which could be a primary problem or secondary to hypoxemia. She first needs to be evaluated for hypoxemia, so a complete blood gas, including co-oximetry, is an initial screening test.

14. This patient's anion gap is 21 mEq/L, indicating a likely anion gap metabolic acidosis. Her venous CO_2 should be about 13 mEq/L, if that is the only acid–base disorder. Her venous CO_2 is, instead, elevated at 35 mEq/L, indicating a coexisting metabolic alkalosis. Patients with electrolytes showing mixed disorders should have blood gases measured to determine if the blood is alkalemic or acidemic, if there are other (respiratory) acid–base disorders, and if oxygenation is adequate.

15. One possible cause of chronic headaches is low-level carbon monoxide poisoning. Neither the arterial blood gas nor the PO_2 rule this out. A blood sample (venous or arterial) should be sent to the blood gas lab for co-oximetry measurement of COHb.

16. The physician, in his concern about possible cardiopulmonary lung disease, has overlooked another common cause of shortness of breath: anemia. The patient's hemoglobin was only 5.8 g/dL, because of excessive menstrual bleeding over several months. Had co-oximetry been done on the blood gas sample, this problem would have been readily uncovered, because Hb content is a co-oximeter measurement. Even without co-oximetry, of course, one should always measure the hemoglobin content in a patient with unexplained dyspnea.

CHAPTER

12

Venous Blood Gases

Beyond "All You Really Need to Know"

Many readers of the first edition wanted more! Specifically, more information about blood gases in critical care situations. All well and good, but the philosophy behind this book is to help you learn blood gas interpretation sufficient for most clinical purposes, i.e., all the information that most clinicians really *need* to know. The preceding chapters should fulfill this goal, so consider this chapter optional. It covers blood gases in mixed venous blood, with emphasis on a few critical care diagnoses: sepsis, severe circulatory failure, cardiopulmonary arrest, and mitochondrial poisoning.

BLOOD GASES IN MIXED VENOUS BLOOD

Our ability to assess oxygenation is usually limited to the whole patient. Apart from some specialized protocols, we are not able to assess oxygenation of individual organs. Specific organ hypoxia is usually recognized only after damage has occurred, e.g., shock liver with elevated liver enzymes and brain ischemia that causes encephalopathy. This situation is unfortunate because some clinical conditions (e.g., septic shock) may cause selective organ hypoxia even though the patient's global oxygen supply appears adequate.

In stable patients with normal mental status and cardiovascular exam (based on the history, physical examination, and chest x-ray), arterial oxygen content (CaO_2) and its components are usually sufficient to assess adequacy of oxygen delivery. However, knowledge of CaO_2 alone may not be sufficient in patients with impaired circulation, e.g., sepsis, shock, and severe congestive heart failure. In these conditions, it may be important to assess oxygenation using the mixed venous oxygen saturation (SvO_2).

Mixed venous blood is blood in the pulmonary artery, the single location where one can be certain that venous return from all the body's organs is thoroughly "mixed." Comparison with arterial blood shows that, except for oxygen pressure and saturation (PO_2 and SO_2, respectively), mixed venous blood gas values are close to those of arterial blood (Table 12.1).

TABLE 12.1. NORMAL BLOOD GAS VALUES IN ARTERIAL AND MIXED VENOUS BLOOD (AT REST)

VALUE	ARTERIAL	MIXED VENOUS	TYPICAL A–V DIFFERENCE
PO_2 (mm Hg)	70–100	35–40	PaO_2 – 60
SO_2 (%)	93–98	65–75	SaO_2 – 25
PCO_2 (mm Hg)	35–45	42–52	6–8
pH	7.35–7.45	7.32–7.41	0.03–0.04
HCO_3^- (mEq/L)	22–26	24–28	2–4

Unlike the values for pH, PCO_2 and HCO_3^-, the difference between arterial and venous *oxygen* values is wide and highly variable. This is one reason why peripheral venous blood can never be used to assess oxygenation, whereas measurements from a free-flowing peripheral venous sample can often be helpful in assessing acid–base status.

A physician draws a radial artery blood sample from a hospitalized patient who is in mild respiratory distress and sends it for blood gas analysis. Because the plunger of the syringe has to be pulled back to obtain the blood, the physician is not sure if he has sampled the artery or the vein. The blood gas values return showing pH = 7.25, PCO_2 = 76 mm Hg, PO_2 = 42 mm Hg, and oxygen saturation = 77%. The physician's reaction is that he must have sent a venous sample because "the patient is not that bad." Assuming this is correct, what could one still conclude from these blood gas values?

In this example, the measured PO_2 and oxygen saturation may be arterial *or* venous; the value for oxygen saturation could (and should) be confirmed with a quick measurement of pulse oximetry. The pH and PCO_2 values, however, are very abnormal and indicate a state of respiratory acidosis *irrespective of the blood's origin,* because venous pH and $PaCO_2$ are usually close to the arterial values. Except in states of severe hypoperfusion, pH and PCO_2 do not share the large differences that exist between arterial (PaO_2 and SaO_2) and venous (PvO_2 and SvO_2) values (Table 12.1). It would be a major pitfall to think that this pH and PCO_2 are venous only because they are so abnormal.

For people breathing room air who are not hemodynamically compromised, venous oxygen values stay in a fairly narrow range (PvO_2 = 35–40 mm Hg, SvO_2 = 65–75%); this is true even when PaO_2 falls to a low level, e.g., down to 50 mm Hg. Venous O_2 is determined mainly by the cardiac output (C.O.) and the amount of oxygen extracted by the tissues, and to a lesser extent by the arterial oxygen pressure, saturation, and content. When PaO_2, SaO_2, or CaO_2 fall, cardiac output and/or oxygen extraction increase to maintain adequate oxygen delivery; as a result, venous oxygen values do not change much, if at all.

OXYGEN DELIVERY, OXYGEN UPTAKE, AND THE FICK EQUATION

To explain this last point further, it will be necessary to introduce two important equations for oxygen delivery and oxygen uptake. Refer to Figure 12.1 as you read through the following paragraphs.

Oxygen delivery

Oxygen delivery is simply the amount of oxygen (in mL O_2/minute) delivered by the circulation. Because the amount of oxygen in the blood is the oxygen

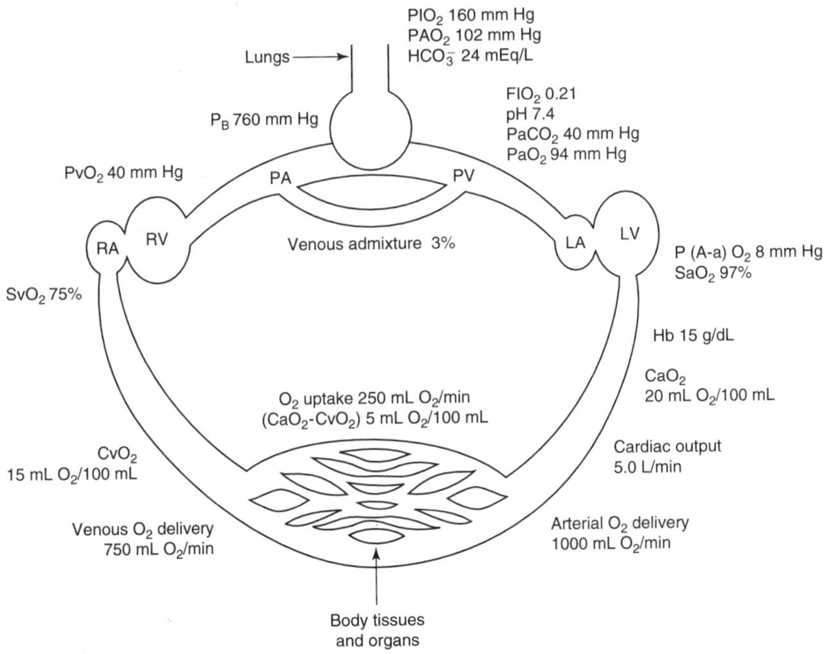

Figure 12.1. Normal arterial and venous oxygen values. A normal pulmonary venous admixture of 3.0% is schematically shown as a shunt between the pulmonary artery and pulmonary venous circulations. *RA*, right atrium; *RV*, right ventricle; *PA*, pulmonary arteries; *PV*, pulmonary veins; *LA*, left atrium; *LV*, left ventricle. Modified from Martin L. Pulmonary physiology in clinical practice. St. Louis: Mosby-Year Book, 1987.

content and the amount of blood delivered is the cardiac output (C.O.), O_2 delivery is simply cardiac output × oxygen content. The equation varies between the arterial and venous circulations only by the difference in oxygen content.

$$\text{Arterial } O_2 \text{ delivery} = \text{C.O.} \times CaO_2$$
$$\text{Venous } O_2 \text{ delivery} = \text{C.O.} \times CvO_2$$

Assuming a normal cardiac output of 5 L/min and arterial oxygen content of 20 mL O_2/dL, O_2 delivery for the arterial circulation is

$$O_2 \text{ delivery} = 5000 \text{ mL } O_2/\text{min} \times 20 \text{ mL } O_2/\text{dL} = 1000 \text{ mL } O_2/\text{min}$$

Oxygen uptake

Oxygen uptake, $\dot{V}O_2$, is the amount of oxygen metabolically used by the body each minute. $\dot{V}O_2$ is simply the difference between arterial O_2 delivery and venous O_2 delivery.

$$\dot{V}O_2 = \text{arterial } O_2 \text{ delivery} - \text{venous } O_2 \text{ delivery}$$

With this idea in mind ,we can easily derive the Fick equation for oxygen delivery as follows:

$$\dot{V}O_2 = (\text{C.O.} \times CaO_2) - (\text{C.O.} \times CvO_2)$$
$$\dot{V}O_2 = \text{C.O.} \times (CaO_2 - CvO_2)$$

This important equation states that the amount of oxygen used by the body each minute is equal to the cardiac output times the difference between arterial and venous oxygen content. Using values for a normal person at rest:

$$\dot{V}O_2 = 5000 \text{ mL/min} \times (20 \text{ mL } O_2/\text{dL} - 15\ O_2/\text{dL}) = 250 \text{ mL } O_2/\text{min}$$

Note that of the 1000 mL O_2 delivered to the tissues per minute, an oxygen uptake ($\dot{V}O_2$) of 250 mL O_2/min is only 25%, leaving a fairly large reserve of oxygen returning to the right side of the heart, 750 mL O_2/min (Fig. 12.1). There is nothing intuitive about the 25% rate of oxygen uptake; it is just the typical percentage used by healthy individuals at rest.

Clinical Problem 12.1. What is the arterial O_2 delivery in each of the following situations?

a. CaO_2 = 12 mL O_2/dL, C.O. = 4 L/min
b. SaO_2 = 100%, Hb = 8 g/dL, C.O. = 6 L/min
c. PaO_2 = 60 mm Hg, pH = 7.40, Hb = 10 g/dL, C.O. = 3 L/min

Clinical Problem 12.2. What is the oxygen uptake in the following situations?

a. C.O. = 6 L/min, SaO_2 = 100%, SvO_2 = 60%, Hb = 10 g/dL
b. C.O. = 4 L/min, CaO_2 = 20 mL O_2/dL, PvO_2 = 27 mm Hg; venous pH = 7.40, Hb = 15 g/dL
c. C.O. = 5 L/min, a–v O_2 difference = 7 mL O_2/dL

$CaO_2 - CvO_2$, or the *a–v O_2 difference,* is an important concept in understanding total body oxygenation. The larger the a–v O_2 difference, the lower the CvO_2 and, therefore, the lower the mixed venous O_2 saturation, SvO_2. A very low SvO_2 usually indicates that the maximum amount of oxygen is being extracted from the tissues and that the patient is in or near a state of anaerobic metabolism. In critically ill patients, unchecked anaerobic metabolism is usually the harbinger of death. In severe circulatory failure, SvO_2 may be critically low even while PaO_2 is adequate; thus SvO_2 can be a more reliable indicator of overall oxygenation.

While normal cardiac output and arterial oxygen content vary appreciably from person to person, the normal resting O_2 extraction of 25% is fairly uniform. An oxygen uptake of 25% leaves a lot of reserve oxygen—75% of the total O_2 delivery—returning to the heart in the venous circulation. There is reason for such a large reserve; it might be needed during exercise or severe illness. Because cardiac output is the same in both the venous and arterial circulation, the venous oxygen delivery (amount of O_2 returning to the right ventricle) is 750 mL O_2/dL (Fig. 12.1). Working backward from this value:

$$\text{Venous } O_2 \text{ delivery} = 750 \text{ mL } O_2\text{/min} = CvO_2 \times 5000 \text{ mL/min}$$

$$CvO_2 = \frac{750 \text{ mL } O_2\text{/min}}{5000 \text{ mL/min}} = 15 \text{ mL } O_2\text{/dL}$$

Because hemoglobin content is also the same in the arterial and venous circulation, and 25% of delivered oxygen is normally extracted by the tissues, it follows that the venous O_2 content will be 75% of arterial content, or 15 mL O_2/min in this example.

COMPENSATION TO MAINTAIN OXYGEN UPTAKE

Adequate oxygen uptake is crucial for survival. When the $\dot{V}O_2$ is threatened, the body will generally make physiologic adaptations to preserve it: increase the cardiac output and/or extract more than 25% of the delivered O_2 (Table 12.2).

Obviously, reduction in either C.O. or CaO_2 can lower oxygen delivery. In either case—reduced C.O. or reduced CaO_2—lactic acidosis and death will ensue if tissue oxygen uptake ($\dot{V}O_2$) is not maintained in some fashion by the product of [C.O. × (CaO_2 − CvO_2)]. It follows from the Fick equation that there are only a few physiologic compensatory mechanisms by which the body can maintain oxygen uptake when it is threatened by decreased oxygen (Table 12.2).

USING SvO_2 TO ASSESS OXYGENATION

Pitfalls in using SvO_2 to assess global oxygenation are both technical and theoretical. Technical problems relate to obtaining a pulmonary artery sample; it requires insertion of a catheter in the patient's pulmonary artery, a procedure not without risk and expense. Assuming a proper mixed venous sample and an accurately measured SvO_2, two statements appear valid in patients at rest:

- An abnormally low SvO_2 indicates inadequate oxygen delivery for the body's needs; the lower the SvO_2, the more severe the inadequacy.
- A normal SvO_2 suggests, but does not guarantee, that oxygenation is adequate.

Abnormally Low SvO_2 Indicates Inadequate Oxygen Delivery

When cardiac output is decreased or cannot be augmented to compensate for a decrease in CaO_2, the mixed venous oxygen content (and thus SvO_2 and PvO_2) *will fall.* Normally, both the cardiac output and the CaO_2 − CvO_2 can increase up to threefold as compensation, i.e., up to 15 L/min for C.O. and 15 mL O_2/100 mL for CaO_2 − CvO_2.

TABLE 12.2. COMPENSATORY MECHANISMS TO MAINTAIN ADEQUATE OXYGEN UPTAKE: EFFECT ON CvO_2, SvO_2, AND PvO_2

PROBLEM	COMPENSATORY MECHANISM	CvO_2, SvO_2, AND PvO_2
Decreased C.O.	Increase in CaO_2 − CvO_2	All reduced
Decreased CaO_2[a]	Increase in C.O.	All normal
	and/or	
	Maintenance of CaO_2 − CvO_2	All reduced

[a]From low SaO_2 or anemia.

Increasing $CaO_2 - CvO_2$ is almost always at the expense of lowering CvO_2. Thus SvO_2 is a barometer of the adequacy of oxygen delivery (C.O. × CaO_2) for the body's overall oxygen needs. (Compensatory mechanisms to raise CaO_2 are limited. Owing to the flattening of the O_2 dissociation curve above a PaO_2 of 60 mm Hg, hyperventilation barely raises SaO_2. Furthermore, any increase in hemoglobin concentration would take a long time to occur.)

When SvO_2 falls to 40% or less (roughly corresponding to a PvO_2 of 27 mm Hg at pH 7.36), the limits of compensation are such that any further fall in SvO_2 will likely result in anaerobic metabolism and lactic acidosis. This condition should be considered preterminal unless reversal is rapid.

Clinical Problem 12.3. Calculate the SvO_2 given the following values. In each case, hemoglobin = 15 gm/dL and CaO_2 = 20 O_2/dL.

a. C.O. = 5 L/min, $\dot{V}O_2$ = 200 mL O_2/min
b. C.O. = 8 L/min, $\dot{V}O_2$ = 300 mL O_2/min
c. C.O. = 2 L/min, $\dot{V}O_2$ = 250 mL O_2/min

Clinical Problem 12.4. Below are baseline values from a patient in the intensive care unit.

Hb = 15 g/dL
SaO_2 = 98%
C.O. = 5 L/min
$\dot{V}O_2$ = 250 mL/min
SvO_2 = 75%

Assuming that $\dot{V}O_2$ stays constant, calculate the resulting SvO_2 for each of the following changes:

a. Hb falls to 10 g/dL
b. SaO_2 decreases to 80%
c. C.O. decreases to 3 L/min

Normal SvO_2 Suggests That Oxygenation Is Adequate

The reasons why a normal SvO_2 suggests, but does not guarantee, that oxygenation is adequate include the following:

- Regional hypoperfusion may be masked by adequate blood flow to the rest of the body. Thus one organ could be oxygen deficient, yet its oxygen-poor venous return may not cause a significant reduction in the mixed venous oxygen content.
- Left-to-right systemic shunts may have the same effect as regional hypoperfusion. These shunts have been described in both septic and hemodynamic shock. If oxygenated blood is shunted from the systemic arteries to the veins (thus bypassing capillaries), a normal (or even elevated) SvO_2 may result. This measurement could be falsely reassuring, because selective tissues or organs may be critically hypoxic and on the verge of irreversible damage.
- In some conditions, such as cyanide poisoning, oxygen delivery is adequate but the mitochondria are poisoned, so that oxygen transfer is blocked between systemic capillaries and the cells. Again, SvO_2 may be normal or even *above normal.* In fact, a high SvO_2 is a diagnostic clue for of cyanide toxicity.

In summary, SvO_2 may be the best *single* measurement by which to assess global adequacy of oxygenation in some critically ill patients. If SvO_2 is reduced, the patient's ability to efficiently oxygenate all organs is either impaired or severely strained. If SvO_2 is normal, oxygenation is probably adequate as long as there is no problem with regional hypoperfusion, left-to-right shunting, or mitochondrial oxygen uptake.

Note that mixed venous PO_2 (PvO_2) can also be used in lieu of SvO_2. Of the two values, however, SvO_2 should be the more reliable because it is solely a function of arterial oxygen delivery and oxygen uptake. In contrast, PvO_2 depends on the SvO_2 *and* on the position of the oxygen dissociation curve.

Venous blood is more acidic than arterial blood; hence the venous oxygen dissociation curve is shifted to the right of the arterial curve. For a given SvO_2, the greater the rightward shift of the curve, the higher the PvO_2. Other factors besides pH can also influence the curve, such as the red cell concentration of 2,3-diphosphoglycerate, so the exact relationship of SvO_2 to PvO_2 cannot be predicted in critically ill patients. If PvO_2 is used to assess oxygenation, it must be measured and not simply estimated from the SvO_2. An SvO_2 of 75% could represent a wide range of PvO_2 values, depending on the position of the oxygen dissociation curve.

Clinical Problem 12.5. What are the SvO_2 and PvO_2 in each of the following situations in a 30-year-old intensive care patient? Assume the patient's lungs, acid–base state, and alveolar–arterial PO_2 difference are normal; barometric pressure is 760 mm Hg.

a. C.O. = 5 L/min, FIO_2 = 0.21, Hb = 15 g/dL, $\dot{V}O_2$ = 250 mL O_2/min, pH = 7.40
b. Same as situation a, *except* C.O. = 2.5 L/min, pH = 7.30
c. Same as situation a, *except* FIO_2 = 1.00, pH = 7.50
d. Same as situation a, *except* Hb = 8 g/dL, pH = 7.30

Obviously, mixed venous oxygen measurements are obtained only on patients in whom there is reason to suspect inadequate oxygen delivery. Even when a right heart catheter is properly inserted, there may also be technical problems in obtaining a sample from the pulmonary artery. Some right heart catheters contain a fiberoptic sensor at the tip that allows for continuous measurement of SvO_2.

Clinical Problem 12.6. A 69-year-old woman with severe congestive heart failure is being treated in the intensive care unit. Because of concern over decreasing urinary output, a right heart catheter is inserted in her pulmonary artery. The following cardiac output and mixed venous oxygen values are obtained along with arterial blood gas measurements:

C.O. = 2.9 L/min	CaO_2 = 14.5 vol %
PaO_2 = 74 mm Hg	SvO_2 = 54%
SaO_2 = 92%	PvO_2 = 26 mm Hg

She is treated with intravenous dobutamine to augment cardiac output; 3 h later, the following measurements are obtained:

C.O. = 3.8 L/min	CaO_2 = 14.5 vol %
PaO_2= 76 mm Hg	SvO_2 = 65%
SaO_2 = 93%	PvO_2 = 34 mm Hg

Do the mixed venous oxygen measurements (SvO_2, PvO_2) reflect the arterial oxygen measurements (PaO_2, SaO_2)? How would you explain the change in her mixed venous oxygen measurements?

Mixed venous oxygen measurements represent a sophisticated attempt to answer the sometimes difficult question about adequacy of overall oxygenation. For the vast majority of patients, however, measurement of arterial blood gases, along with the physical examination and the clinical course, will be sufficient to assess oxygenation.

VENOUS BLOOD GASES IN CARDIOPULMONARY ARREST

Research on venous blood gases in cardiopulmonary arrest has not only enhanced our understanding of this most critical of all conditions but also contributed to a change in recommended therapy: the elimination of routine intravenous bicarbonate in cardiopulmonary resuscitation (CPR).

Up until the mid-1980s it was routine to give sodium bicarbonate in CPR. The reasoning was that, because lactic acidosis is invariably present during cardiac arrest, the chance for successful resuscitation (including cardiac defibrillation) would be enhanced by buffering lactic acid.

Not much thought was given to the venous blood gases until an important study by Weil et al. (1986). The authors showed a marked disparity between arterial and venous blood gas measurements in intubated patients during cardiac arrest. During CPR, the arterial pH averaged 7.41 and PCO_2, 32 mm Hg, indicating metabolic acidosis and respiratory alkalosis. The mixed venous pH, however, averaged 7.15 and PCO_2, 74 mm Hg. Venous respiratory acidosis in the face of arterial respiratory alkalosis has been termed the venoarterial paradox.

This human study confirmed earlier animal work. During cardiopulmonary arrest and resuscitation in pigs, Weil et al. (1986) had found a "striking difference" in acid–base between arterial (pH = 7.56, $PaCO_2$ = 21 mm Hg) and mixed venous (pH = 7.29, $PaCO_2$ = 54 mm Hg) circulations. Thus both animal and human studies confirmed that in CPR there is a mixed venous respiratory acidosis, whereas arterial blood reflects a respiratory alkalosis.

The authors concluded that mixed venous blood

> most accurately reflects the acid–base state during cardiopulmonary resuscitation, especially the rapid increase in PCO_2. Arterial blood does not reflect the marked reduction in mixed venous (and therefore tissue) pH, and thus arterial blood gases may fail as appropriate guides for acid–based management in this emergency.

The explanation for the venoarterial paradox lies in the fact that the lungs are poorly perfused during CPR; the bulk of the carbon dioxide production is not delivered to the alveoli for gas exchange. The $PaCO_2$ is low because the patient is being manually ventilated, but the only washout of CO_2 occurs in the arterial side of the circulation. In essence there is a backup of CO_2 in the venous circulation, and this backup is not reflected in the arterial circulation. Hence the arterial blood gases don't reflect the venous side.

This understanding brought about a change in the recommendation of sodium bicarbonate for CPR. The drug is no longer recommended as routine therapy in CPR, because the CO_2 generated by the bicarbonate is not ventilated off and ends up only worsening the venous respiratory acidosis. (Furthermore, sodium bicarbonate does not improve the chances of successful defibrillation.)

The venoarterial paradox also helps explain an observation mentioned in Chapter 3: end-tidal PCO_2 ($PetCO_2$) falls precipitously in cardiac arrest, and its return toward normal signals a return of circulation. The reason is that with manual or mechanical ventilation during CPR all the PCO_2 in the pulmonary capillaries is quickly washed out, leaving the alveolar PCO_2 very low, usually < 10 mm Hg. Because very little new CO_2 from metabolism is delivered to the pulmonary circulation, alveolar and hence end-tidal PCO_2 remain very low until there is a return of circulation.

SUMMARY: VENOUS BLOOD GASES

In summary, venous blood gases can extend our understanding of oxygenation and help clarify acid–base and ventilatory status in some critical care situations. Although this information may not be necessary for most clinicians interested in routine blood gas interpretation, it is nonetheless interesting and informative.

Clinical Problem 12.7. For each of the following situations, state whether you would expect to find SvO_2 in the normal range, or higher or lower than normal.

a. Cardiac arrest with resuscitation efforts lasting 10 min
b. Anemia, Hb=10 g/dL
c. Extreme exercise, with cardiac output 2.5 times normal
d. Hypoxemia, PaO_2 on room air = 60 mm Hg
e. Mitochondrial poisoning from cyanide, with elevated blood lactate level
f. Carbon monoxide poisoning, COHb = 50%
g. Acute respiratory acidosis, pH = 7.30, $PaCO_2$ = 55 mm Hg

ANSWERS TO CLINICAL PROBLEMS

12.1.

Situation a:

$$\begin{aligned} O_2 \text{ delivery} &= CaO_2 \times \text{C.O.} \\ &= 12 \text{ mL } O_2/\text{dL} \times 4 \text{ L/min} \\ &= 480 \text{ mL } O_2/\text{min} \end{aligned}$$

Situation b: First, calculate CaO_2:

$$CaO_2 = (1.00 \times 8 \times 1.34) + 0.003\,(600) = 12.5 \text{ mL } O_2/\text{dL}$$

Then

$$\begin{aligned} O_2 \text{ delivery} &= CaO_2 \times \text{C.O.} \\ &= 12.5\text{mL } O_2/\text{dL} \times 6 \text{ L/min} = 750 \text{ mL } O_2/\text{min} \end{aligned}$$

Situation c: Because SaO_2 is not provided, it should be calculated from the PaO_2 of 60 mm Hg. Assuming no abnormal hemoglobin binding, SaO_2 is ~ 90% at a pH of 7.4. Ignoring the small contribution from PO_2,

$$\begin{aligned} CaO_2 &= 0.90 \times 1.34 \times 10 = 12.06 \text{ mL } O_2/\text{dL} \\ O_2 \text{ delivery} &= 12.06 \text{ mL } O_2/\text{dL} \times 3 \text{ L/min} = 361.8 \text{ mL } O_2/\text{min} \end{aligned}$$

12.2.

Situation a:

$$\begin{aligned} \dot{V}O_2 &= \text{C.O.} \times (CaO_2 - CvO_2) \\ &= 6 \text{ L/min } [(1.00 \times 1.34 \times 10) - (0.60 \times 1.34 \times 10)] \\ &= 6000 \text{ mL/min} \times 5.4 \text{ mL } O_2/\text{dL} \\ &= 324 \text{ mL } O_2/\text{min} \end{aligned}$$

Situation b: The venous oxygen saturation is determined from the venous PO_2, which is 27 mm Hg; this gives a saturation of 50% at pH of 7.4. Thus

$$\begin{aligned} \dot{V}O_2 &= 4 \text{ L/min } [20 - (0.50 \times 1.34 \times 15)] \\ &= 4000 \text{ mL/min} \times 10 \text{ mL } O_2/\text{dL} \\ &= 400 \text{ mL } O_2/\text{min} \end{aligned}$$

Situation c:

$$\dot{V}O_2 = 5 \text{ L/min} \times 7 \text{ mL } O_2/\text{dL} = 350 \text{ mL } O_2/\text{min}$$

12.3.

Situation a:

$$\begin{aligned} \dot{V}O_2 &= \text{C.O.} \times (CaO_2 - CvO_2) \\ 200 \text{ mL } O_2/\text{min} &= 5 \text{ L/min} \times (CaO_2 - CvO_2) \end{aligned}$$

$$CaO_2 - CvO_2 = \frac{200 \text{ mL } O_2/\text{min}}{5 \text{ L/min}} = 5 \text{ mL } O_2/\text{dL}$$

$$\text{Since } CaO_2 = 20 \text{ mL } O_2/dL$$
$$(CaO_2 - CvO_2) = 5 \text{mL } O_2/dL,$$
$$\text{and } CvO_2 = 15 \text{ mL } O_2/dL = SvO_2 \times 1.34 \times 15$$
$$SvO_2 = 75\%$$

Situation b:

$$\dot{V}O_2 = C.O. \times (CaO_2 - CvO_2)$$
$$300 \text{ mL } O_2/\text{min} = 8 \text{ L/min} \times (CaO_2 - CvO_2)$$
$$CaO_2 - CvO_2 = \frac{300 \text{ mL } O_2/\text{min}}{8 \text{ L/min}} = 3.75 \text{ mL } O_2/dL$$
$$\text{Since } CaO_2 = 20 \text{ mL } O_2/dL,$$
$$\text{and } (CaO_2 - CvO_2) = 3.75 \text{ mL } O_2/dL,$$

$$CvO_2 = 16.25 \text{ mL } O_2/dL = SvO_2 \times 1.34 \times 15$$
$$SvO_2 = 81\%$$

Situation c.

$$\dot{V}O_2 = C.O. \times (CaO_2 - CvO_2)$$
$$250 \text{ mL } O_2/\text{min} = 2 \text{ L/min} \times (CaO_2 - CvO_2)$$
$$CaO_2 - CvO_2 = \frac{250 \text{ mL } O_2/\text{min}}{2 \text{ L/min}} = 12.5 \text{ mL } O_2/dL$$

$$\text{Since } CaO_2 = 20 \text{ mL } O_2/dL \text{ and}$$
$$(CaO_2 - CvO_2) = 12.5 \text{ mL } O_2/dL$$
$$CvO_2 = 7.5 \text{ mL } O_2/dL = SvO_2 \times 1.34 \times 15$$
$$SvO_2 = 37\%$$

12.4.

Situation a:

$$CaO_2 = 10 \times 1.34 \times 0.98 = 13.1 \text{ mL } O_2/dL$$
$$\dot{V}O_2 = 250 \text{ mL } O_2/\text{min} = 5 \text{ L/min} \times (CaO_2 - CvO_2)$$

$$CaO_2 - CvO_2 = 5 \text{ mL } O_2/dL$$
$$CvO_2 = 13.1 - 5 = 8.1 \text{ mL } O_2/dL$$

$$8.1 \text{ mL } O_2/dL = SvO_2 \times 1.34 \times 10$$
$$SvO_2 = 60\%$$

Situtation b:

$$CaO_2 = 15 \times 1.34 \times 0.80 = 16.1 \text{ mL } O_2/dL$$
$$\dot{V}O_2 = 250 \text{ mL } O_2/min = 5 \text{ L/min} \times (CaO_2 - CvO_2)$$
$$CaO_2 - CvO_2 = 5 \text{ mL } O_2/dL$$
$$CvO_2 = 16.1 - 5 = 11.1 \text{ mL } O_2/dL$$
$$11.1 \text{ mL } O_2/dL = SvO_2 \times 1.34 \times 15$$
$$SvO_2 = 55\%$$

Situation c:

$$CaO_2 = 15 \times 1.34 \times 0.98 = 19.7 \text{ mL } O_2/dL$$
$$\dot{V}O_2 = 250 \text{ mL } O_2/min = 3 \text{ L/min} \times (CaO_2 - CvO_2)$$
$$CaO_2 - CvO_2 = 8.3 \text{ mL } O_2/dL$$
$$CvO_2 = 19.7 - 8.3 = 11.4 \text{ mL } O_2/dL$$
$$11.4 \text{ mL } O_2/dL = SvO_2 \times 1.34 \times 15$$
$$SvO_2 = 57\%$$

12.5.

Situation a:

Since Hb = 15 gm/dL and the lungs are normal at sea level, then the PaO_2 is ~ 100 mm Hg and the SaO_2 is ~ 98%; hence

$$CaO_2 = (15 \times 1.34 \times 0.98) + 0.003\,(100) = 20 \text{ mL } O_2/dL$$
$$\dot{V}O_2 = 250 \text{ mL } O_2/min = 5 \text{ L/min} \times (CaO_2 - CvO_2)$$

$$CaO_2 - CvO_2 = 5 \text{ mL } O_2/dL$$
$$CaO_2 = 20 \text{ mL } O_2/dL$$
$$CvO_2 = 15 \text{ mL } O_2/dL = 15 \times 1.34 \times SvO_2$$

$$SvO_2 = \frac{15}{15 \times 1.34} = 75\%$$

$$PvO_2 = \sim 40 \text{ mm Hg}$$

Situation b:

$$CaO_2 = (15 \times 1.34 \times 0.98) + 0.003\,(100) = 20 \text{ mL } O_2/dL$$
$$\dot{V}O_2 = 250 \text{ mL } O_2/min = 2.5 \text{ L/min} \times (CaO_2 - CvO_2)$$
$$CaO_2 - CvO_2 = 10 \text{ mL } O_2/dL$$
$$CaO_2 = 20 \text{ mL } O_2/dL$$
$$CvO_2 = 10 \text{ mL } O_2/dL$$

$$10 \text{ mL } O_2/dL = 15 \times 1.34 \times SvO_2$$

$$SvO_2 = \frac{10}{15 \times 1.34} = 50\%$$

$$PvO_2 = \sim 29 \text{ mm Hg}$$

Situation c:

$$CaO_2 = (15 \times 1.34 \times 1) + 0.003\ (600) = 21.9 \text{ mL } O_2/dL$$
$$\dot{V}O_2 = 250 \text{ mL } O_2/\text{min} = 5 \text{ L/min} \times (CaO_2 - CvO_2)$$
$$CaO_2 - CvO_2 = 5 \text{ mL } O_2/dL$$

$$CaO_2 = 21.9 \text{ mL } O_2/dL$$
$$CvO_2 = 16.9 \text{ mL } O_2/dL$$
$$16.9 \text{ mL } O_2/dL = 15 \times 1.34 \times SvO_2$$

$$SvO_2 = \frac{16.9}{15 \times 1.34} = 84\%$$

$$PvO_2 = \sim 55 \text{ mm Hg}$$

Situation d:

$$CaO_2 = (7.8 \times 1.34 \times 0.98) + 0.003\ (100) = 10.8 \text{ mL } O_2/dL$$
$$\dot{V}O_2 = 250 \text{ mL } O_2/\text{min} = 5 \text{ L/min} \times (CaO_2 - CvO_2)$$

$$CaO_2 - CvO_2 = 5 \text{ mL } O_2/dL$$
$$CaO_2 = 10.8 \text{ mL } O_2/dL$$
$$CvO_2 = 5.8 \text{ mL } O_2/dL$$
$$5.8 \text{ mL } O_2/dL = 8 \times 1.34 \times SvO_2$$

$$SvO_2 = \frac{5.8}{8 \times 1.34} = 54\%$$

$$PvO_2 = \sim 30 \text{ mm Hg}$$

12.6. The mixed venous oxygen measurements (SvO_2, PvO_2) do not reflect the arterial measurements. Here the arterial oxygen measurements change very little, whereas the mixed venous measurements increase with the addition of dobutamine. Clearly, the increase in cardiac output (from 2.9 to 3.8 L/min) has improved overall oxygenation, but you wouldn't know it from the arterial measurements alone.

12.7.

a. Lower
b. Normal
c. Lower
d. Normal
e. Higher
f. Lower
g. Normal

CHAPTER

13

Pitfalls in Blood Gas Interpretation

As with any lab result, there are potential pitfalls in interpreting blood gas data. This chapter briefly discusses the most common pitfalls, which span the range from sampling errors to ignoring valid data. It is beyond the scope of this book to present techniques of drawing and analyzing the arterial blood sample, but these aspects should be recognized as the source of potential errors in interpretation. Several excellent texts cover technical and methodologic aspects in detail, and I recommend them to interested readers (see Appendix E). Here are 15 common pitfalls in blood gas interpretation.

1. **Not an arterial sample.** Sometimes there is no way to know if blood gas data are from an arterial or venous blood sample. The person drawing the sample can usually tell the difference. If blood pulsates into the syringe and the syringe plunger rises on its own, the sample is most likely arterial; venous pressure is seldom sufficient to fill a syringe on its own. Conversely, if the syringe can be filled only by manually pulling on the plunger *and* the PaO_2 is very low, the sample is likely venous. Peripheral vein PO_2 is almost always < 40 and often < 30 mm Hg. A PO_2 value > 40 mm Hg or an oxygen saturation $> 75\%$ is most likely *not* from a pure venous sample. Unlike venous PO_2 and O_2 saturation, venous pH and PCO_2 are often close to arterial values (see Table 12.1), so abnormal pH and PCO_2 *cannot* be used to classify any blood gas data as venous in origin (see Chapter 12).

   On occasion, there is venous admixture; the sample contains some venous blood and, therefore, a lower PO_2 than would be found in pure arterial blood. Venous admixture is more likely to occur with multiple passes of the syringe needle and also when the femoral artery is sampled, because this vessel is adjacent to the large-capacity femoral vein. A single puncture with rapid filling helps ensure against sample contamination. When in doubt about the validity of a blood sample, the test should be repeated or a pulse oximetry measurement obtained instead.

2. **Patient not in a steady state.** Before blood gas data are used for patient management, the patient should be in a steady state in terms of oxygenation and ventilation. This pitfall can occur if the blood sample is from a patient recently connected to a mechanical ventilator or changed to a new FIO_2. It takes only about 3 min for people with healthy lungs to achieve a steady state when the FIO_2 is changed (as when receiving supplemental oxygen). Patients with chronic airways obstruction may take up to 20 min to reach a steady state. As a general rule, wait at least 20 min before drawing a blood sample if there has been a change in FIO_2. In mechanically-ventilated patients, in whom both $PaCO_2$ and PaO_2 may be affected after a change in ventilator settings, wait at least 30 min for the patient to reach a steady state.
3. **Sample syringe contains too much anticoagulant.** Several studies have analyzed the effects of anticoagulant on blood gas data. The effect depends on the type of anticoagulant (most commonly lithium heparin, sometimes sodium heparin), its concentration (1000, 5000, and 25000 units/mL), and the ratio of anticoagulant volume to blood volume in the syringe. Heparin is the most commonly used anticoagulant; an excess in the syringe causes a drop in $PaCO_2$. This problem seems to occur most frequently when blood is drawn from an indwelling arterial line. Such lines are routinely flushed with a heparin solution; failure to discard the first few milliliters of aspirated blood will give excess heparin in the sample.

   The pH change from excess anticoagulant is variable because heparin has a slightly acidic pH, offsetting any rise in blood pH when $PaCO_2$ falls. Because of all the variables, if too much heparin is used one can't reliably determine true blood gas values from the measured data. If the syringe is part of a commercial kit, follow the manufacturer's recommendations about how much anticoagulant to leave in the barrel. Otherwise, it is best to wet the inside of the syringe and needle with heparin and leave no visible accumulation before drawing blood.
4. **Sample contains an air bubble or the sample has been left open to air.** At sea level, the atmospheric PO_2 is about 160 mm Hg (0.21×760 mm Hg). If the patient's PaO_2 is < 160 mm Hg and the sample contains an air bubble, or the syringe is left open to air, the PO_2 in the sample will rise. The degree of rise depends on the initial PaO_2 and how long the sample is exposed to air. Exposure of the sample to air is one possible explanation for a negative $P(A\text{–}a)O_2$. Conversely, if the patient's true PaO_2 is > 160 mm Hg, the exposed sample's PO_2 will fall. Because ambient air contains almost no CO_2, the resulting $PaCO_2$ of any air-exposed sample can be expected to fall and the resulting pH, to rise.

Occasionally, an air bubble enters the blood gas machine's intake tube and causes erroneous measurement. One result could be an apparent negative $P(A–a)O_2$. If a portion of the blood sample is also run independently in a co-oximeter, the problem can usually be diagnosed. For example, suppose a patient breathing room air has PaO_2 = 149 mm Hg, measured SaO_2 = 82%, and normal %COHb and %MetHb. One likely reason for the falsely high PaO_2 is an air bubble in the blood gas machine tubing that connects to the PaO_2 electrode.

5. **Sample not placed on ice.** Arterial blood samples should always be placed in a bag or container filled with ice before transport to the blood gas lab. Metabolizing blood cells alter blood gas values, principally PaO_2, quickly at normal body temperature (37°C), but much less so at 0°C (temperature of ice water). An iced sample should remain stable for at least 1 h. Any sample not placed in ice should be tested within minutes after it is drawn, or otherwise discarded. The main effect of cellular metabolism is to decrease PO_2. Several studies have shown a remarkable fall in PaO_2 if the blood contains > 100,000 white blood cells/mm^3 (leukocyte larceny), even when the sample is on ice. A white cell count of this magnitude (usually in leukemia) should mandate special handling, i.e., running the sample immediately. Alternatively, check the patient's oxygen saturation by pulse oximetry, which is not affected by extreme leukocytosis (Sacchetti et al. 1990).
6. **Incorrect FIO_2.** Blood gases are usually reported with the FIO_2 entered on the report form. If the FIO_2 is incorrect, the blood gas data may make sense physiologically but be interpreted incorrectly. For example, if a patient is noted to be receiving "40% oxygen by face mask," but the mask was actually off the patient when the blood was drawn, oxygenation may seem worse than it actually is. Another example, fortunately less common, is when the patient is wearing the prescribed oxygen appliance, but the oxygen is disconnected or turned off at the source. Whenever PaO_2 is unexpectedly reduced in a patient receiving supplemental oxygen, the O_2 source should be checked.
7. **Calculated SaO_2 interpreted as measured SaO_2.** This pitfall, extensively discussed in Chapter 5, is easy to avoid if you know how the blood gas lab reports SaO_2. Ideally, the lab should either *not* report a calculated SaO_2 or else note that the reported value represents a calculation and not an actual measurement. The person interpreting the data then has to realize that the calculated SaO_2 may be significantly higher than true (measured) SaO_2 in states of carbon monoxide poisoning and methemoglobinemia (see Chapter 6).

8. **Data physiologically incorrect.** This pitfall occurs when data violate normal human physiology, e.g., the data lead to a negative $P(A\text{–}a)O_2$ or a calculated bicarbonate value impossible to obtain from the measured $PaCO_2$ and pH. The origin of the former problem is usually an FIO_2 listed as room air when the patient is actually receiving supplemental oxygen (compare with Pitfall 6, which is the opposite problem). A physiologically incorrect bicarbonate is usually traceable to a transcription error. For example, if a technician writes down "pH = 7.42, $PaCO_2$ = 38, HCO_3^- = 34," you should immediately recognize a probable transcription error for HCO_3^- and not make any interpretation based on its spuriously high value.
9. **Confusion over effect of patient's temperature.** Arterial blood is always analyzed at normal body temperature, 37°C, in the blood gas machine. If the patient is febrile, the measured PaO_2 and $PaCO_2$ will be *lower* than in the patient; gas molecules are slowed by the lower temperature of the machine and register less pressure. Conversely, if the patient is hypothermic, the measured PaO_2 and $PaCO_2$ will be *higher* than in the patient; gas molecules are speeded up by the higher temperature of the machine and register greater pressure. For each degree centigrade above or below 37°C, the change in PaO_2 is approximately 5 mm Hg and the change in $PaCO_2$, approximately 2 mm Hg. Thus a patient febrile to 39°C, whose measured PaO_2 and $PaCO_2$ are 80 and 40 mm Hg, respectively, has a true or *in vivo* PaO_2 of 90 mm Hg and $PaCO_2$ of 44 mm Hg.

   Although some labs automatically correct for patient temperature, most labs purposely do not correct. On balance, most physicians seem to feel that temperature correction is not necessary and that all blood gas data should be interpreted with reference to normal values at 37°C. It may also be true that a low PaO_2 in a hypothermic patient is just as adequate (because of decreased metabolism) as a normal PaO_2 in an afebrile patient.

   In truth, we don't know what blood gas values "should be" when body temperature is abnormal. The pitfall is not in ignoring patient temperature for purposes of blood gas interpretation, but in making too much of the temperature correction. For most clinical purposes it is best not to bother with any correction. If data are already corrected don't convert back but continue to interpret the data based on normal reference values.

   Finally, it is important to make sure that sequential blood gases in a given patient are all handled the same way. If temperature correction is done for some arterial blood samples and not for others, a change in PaO_2, for example, may reflect only the correction and not any real change in the patient's condition.

10. **Data reported under wrong name or ID number.** This pitfall is easy to avoid if there are previous blood gas results and the current data are way out of line or they don't fit the clinical picture (see Pitfall 12). The pitfall is difficult to avoid if there are no previous blood gas data and the results seem to fit your patient, but really belong to someone else.
11. **Verbal report incorrect.** Sometimes people misremember blood gas data, then report incorrect information to another caregiver. A physician on a busy service might remember three sets of blood gas data but confuse which set goes with which patient. The incorrectly reported data may make sense physiologically and even fit the clinical picture; but because the data belong to some other patient, the wrong treatment is ordered. Anyone responsible for treatment based on blood gas data should make sure the data are accurate. This means not relying on verbal reports that are based on memory.
12. **Data don't fit the clinical picture.** Although one cannot determine blood gas values clinically, sometimes data are clearly way out of line for the clinical status. For example, a report of pH = 7.21 and $PaCO_2$ = 23 mm Hg should be suspect if the patient is alert, in no apparent respiratory distress, and without any clinical disease to explain severe metabolic acidosis. If the data make no clinical sense the test should be repeated. The opposite pitfall may also be encountered (see Pitfall 13).
13. **Correct data are ignored.** This pitfall occurs when the data seem so abnormal for the patient that the physician assumes a lab or sampling error, but the data are in fact accurate. For example, PaO_2 *may* be very low even though the patient is not dyspneic at rest. In such cases, one should not assume a lab or sampling error but either repeat the blood gas test or measure the patient's SaO_2 with pulse oximetry. As with all lab tests, one must use experience and clinical judgment to decide which tests to believe, which to ignore, and which to repeat.
14. **Treating blood gases, not the patient.** A variation of Pitfall 12 occurs when the physician tries to correct the blood gas values with an unneeded treatment. The most common example is intubating a patient with severe respiratory acidosis who is alert and who will likely respond to less invasive therapy. Alert patients with severely abnormal blood gases usually do not need emergent intubation. "Intubate patients, not blood gases" is a useful maxim in these situations. Obviously, avoiding this pitfall is a matter of experience and clinical judgment. Always consider the blood gas values in clinical context and consider how therapy of the basic disease may improve the numbers.

15. **Not obtaining blood gas measurements when indicated.** This is not a pitfall in blood gas interpretation, but instead results from not appreciating when the clinical evaluation necessitates blood gases, i.e., when you need some measurement to assess oxygenation, ventilation, and/or acid–base status. Helping you avoid this pitfall is the focus of Chapter 11.

APPENDIX

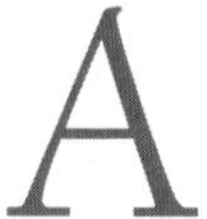

Post-Test

If you mark over 90% correct responses on this post-test, chances are you have learned all you really need to know about arterial blood gas interpretation. Congratulations!

Directions: For each of the following 10 numbered statements or questions, **there may be none, one, or more than one correct response.** Circle the letter next to the correct response(s) *before* checking the answers in Appendix B.

1. Carbon monoxide
   a. Shifts the O_2 dissociation curve to the left
   b. Lowers the PaO_2
   c. Increases the P_{50}
   d. Lowers the CaO_2
   e. Poisoning is treated with a high FIO_2

2. A patient with $PaCO_2 = 75$ mm Hg and $HCO_3^- = 23$ mEq/L most likely has
   a. Acute respiratory acidosis as an isolated primary acid–base disorder
   b. Respiratory acidosis plus metabolic acidosis
   c. A $PaO_2 < 70$ mm Hg if the blood gas was obtained while the patient was breathing room air
   d. A low arterial pH
   e. A low serum sodium

3. Pulse oximetry is generally not accurate in patients
   a. With carbon monoxide intoxication
   b. With poor perfusion of extremities
   c. Of African-American descent
   d. Who are acutely hyperventilating
   e. Who are receiving supplemental oxygen

4. Which of the following statements about hemoglobin is(are) correct?
   a. Oxidized hemoglobin contains iron in the 3^+ or oxidized state and cannot bind oxygen
   b. Deoxygenated hemoglobin contains iron in the 2^+ or ferrous state and is unbound to oxygen
   c. Oxygenated hemoglobin contains iron in the 2^+ or ferrous state and is bound to oxygen
   d. Carboxyhemoglobin contains iron in the 2^+ or ferrous state but not in the 3^+ or ferric state
   e. An SaO_2 of 95% means that 95% of the heme binding sites are bound with oxygen

5. A 49-year-old alcoholic is admitted to hospital after 3 days of vomiting. Arterial blood gas and electrolyte values (on room air) show

pH = 7.50	Na^+ = 138 mEq/L
$PaCO_2$ = 53 mm Hg	K^+ = 2.3 mEq/L
PaO_2 = 55 mm Hg	CO_2 = 42 mEq/L
SaO_2 = 88%	Cl^- = 74 mEq/L

   Which of the following disorder(s) is(are) likely present?
   a. Metabolic acidosis
   b. Metabolic alkalosis
   c. Respiratory alkalosis
   d. Respiratory acidosis
   e. Ventilation–perfusion imbalance

6. A 65-year-old patient with severe emphysema is sitting in bed, breathing at a respiratory rate of 23/min. Arterial blood gas values at this time show

pH = 7.35	SaO_2 = 78%
$PaCO_2$ = 65 mm Hg	Hb = 10 g/dL
PaO_2 = 45 mm Hg	FIO_2 = 0.21

   Which one of the following problem(s) reasonably explain(s) the patient's reduced oxygen content?
   a. Ventilation–perfusion imbalance
   b. Anemia
   c. Excess carbon monoxide
   d. Hypercapnia
   e. Left shift of the oxygen dissociation curve

7. In the clinical setting, which of the following is(are) valid concerning blood gas physiology?
   a. End-tidal PCO_2 should always be higher than arterial PCO_2
   b. Alveolar PO_2 should always be higher than arterial PO_2
   c. Percent oxyhemoglobin + percent carboxyhemoglobin + percent methemoglobin should never exceed 100%
   d. The ratio of dead space to tidal volume should never exceed 1.0
   e. The average airway pressure does not exceed barometric pressure in a spontaneously breathing patient

8. Which of the following is(are) correct about PaO_2?
   a. If the lungs and heart are normal, then PaO_2 is affected only by factors that affect alveolar PO_2
   b. In a person with normal heart and lungs, anemia should not affect PaO_2
   c. PaO_2 will go up in a patient with hemolysis of red blood cells, as oxygen is given off when the cells lyse
   d. As the oxygen dissociation curve shifts to the left, PaO_2 falls because more oxygen becomes bound to hemoglobin
   e. The reason PaO_2 falls with increasing altitude is because the FIO_2 falls

9. In a cup of water at sea level, which of the following statements is(are) correct?
   a. The PaO_2 is the same as in the air above the cup
   b. The $PaCO_2$ is the same as in the air above the cup
   c. The PN_2 is the same as in the air above the cup
   d. The SaO_2 is zero because there is no hemoglobin present
   e. The CaO_2 is zero because there is no hemoglobin present

10. Below are a set of serum electrolytes. State which, if any, of the blood gas measurements could fit with this set of electrolytes.

    Na^+ = 150 mEq/L
    K^+ = 4.3 mEq/L
    CO_2 = 24 mEq/L
    Cl^- = 100 mEq/L

    a. pH = 7.20
    b. pH = 7.50
    c. $PaCO_2$ = 78 mm Hg
    d. pH = 7.23, $PaCO_2$ = 15 mm Hg, PaO_2 = 106 mm Hg
    e. pH = 7.40, PCO_2 = 20 mm Hg, PaO_2 = 67 mm Hg

APPENDIX

B

Answers

ANSWERS TO THE PRE-TEST

1. a, b are correct

   Incorrect:

   c. Patient may hyperventilate by breathing deeper than normal, or may even hyperventilate with both normal rate and depth if the level of CO_2 production falls.

   d. Patient could have metabolic acidosis.

   e. Patient is not in a steady state for gas exchange since there is acute hyperventilation.

2. a, b, c, e are correct

   Incorrect:

   d. In patients who may have lung disease, there are no useful bedside parameters for determining whether $PaCO_2$ is high or low.

3. b, c, e are correct.

   Incorrect:

   a. Anemia reduces oxygen content, not PaO_2.

   d. Carbon monoxide reduces SaO_2 and CaO_2, not PaO_2.

4. a, d are correct

   Incorrect:

   b, c, e. You need at least two of the three variables in the Henderson–Hasselbalch equation to assess the acid–base state of a patient's blood.

5. a, b, c, d are correct

   Incorrect:

   e. In theory, the plasma HCO_3^- calculated from blood gases should be 2–4 mEq/L less than the serum CO_2 measured on a venous sample, because venous bicarbonate is higher than arterial and also because serum CO_2 measurement includes the quantity contributed by dissolved CO_2.

6. a, c, d, e are correct.

   Incorrect:

   b. Other determinants are those factors that affect the position of the oxygen dissociation curve, e.g., temperature, pH, $PaCO_2$, 2,3 DPG.

7. c, d and e are correct

   Incorrect:

   a. Each gram of hemoglobin can combine with 1.34 mL of O_2.
   b. Normal CaO_2 is between 16 and 22 mL O_2/dL.

8. a, c, e are correct

   Incorrect:

   b. Arterial PO_2 and pH are not directly related by any equation.
   d. Arterial PO_2 is related to SaO_2 by the O_2 dissociation curve, which has a sigmoid configuration.

9. b, d are correct

   Incorrect:

   a. *Hyperventilation* and *hypoventilation* should only be used clinically as they relate to the $PaCO_2$.
   c. People with normal lungs can increase arterial PO_2 above 100 mm Hg with hyperventilation.
   e. A patient can have profound acid–base imbalance yet normal pH from opposing acid–base disorders (e.g., combined metabolic acidosis and metabolic alkalosis).

10. a, b, e are correct

   Incorrect:

   c. The pulse oximeter is *not* equal in accuracy to the co-oximeter, because the latter employs four wavelengths of light to differentiate hemoglobin moieties; the pulse oximeter uses only two wavelengths, and reads carboxyhemoglobin and oxyhemoglobin together.
   d. The end-tidal PCO_2 is usually equal to or *lower* than the $PaCO_2$. In lung diseases with V–Q imbalance, excess dead space contributes air with low or zero PCO_2 to the end-tidal sample, making end-tidal PCO_2 lower than $PaCO_2$.

ANSWERS TO THE POST-TEST

1. a, d, e are correct
   Incorrect:
   b. PaO_2 is not affected.
   c. The P_{50} is lower because CO shifts the curve to the left.

2. b, c, d are correct
   Incorrect:
   a. The slightly lowered bicarbonate points to a metabolic acidosis.
   e. There is no predictable correlation between serum sodium and acid–base state.

3. a, b are correct
   Incorrect:
   c, d, e, Skin pigment, acute hyperventilation, and supplemental oxygen should not affect SaO_2 readings with modern pulse oximeters.

4. All are correct

5. a, b, d, e are correct
   Incorrect:
   c. The patient is hypoventilating, not hyperventilating, as would be the case with respiratory alkalosis.

6. a, b, d are correct
   Incorrect:
   c. The SaO_2 of 78% is appropriate for a PaO_2 of 45 mm Hg and pH of 7.35. These values do not suggest the presence of excess carbon monoxide.
   e. With a low pH and high $PaCO_2$, the oxygen dissociation curve would be shifted to the right.

7. b, c, d, e are correct
   Incorrect:
   a. End-tidal PCO_2 should always be equal to or *lower* than the arterial PCO_2.

8. a and b are correct
   Incorrect:
   c. There is rapid equilibration with the atmosphere of any released oxygen molecules and PaO_2 will not increase.

d. Shift of the oxygen dissociation curve affects oxygen saturation, not PaO_2.
e. FIO_2 is constant throughout the breathable atmosphere; the barometric pressure falls with altitude.

9. a, b, c, d are correct.
   Incorrect:
   e. CaO_2 is not zero because dissolved oxygen is present.

10. a, b, c are correct.
    Incorrect:
    d. A low pH and $PaCO_2$ will give a low CO_2, not a normal value of 24 mEq/L.
    e. A normal pH and low $PaCO_2$ will give a low CO_2, not a normal value of 24 mEq/L.

APPENDIX

C

Symbols and Abbreviations

A	=	Alveolar
a	=	Arterial
AG	=	Anion gap
ΔAG	=	Delta anion gap; difference between measured and normal AG
ABG	=	Arterial blood gas
BB	=	Buffer base
BG	=	Bicarbonate gap
BE	=	Base excess
BUN	=	Blood urea nitrogen, an index of renal function
CaO_2	=	Content of oxygen in arterial blood, in mL O_2/dL
Cl^-	=	Chloride ion
CO	=	Carbon monoxide
CO_2	=	Carbon dioxide; CO_2 is symbol for both CO_2 as a blood gas (measured as PCO_2, in mm Hg) and for the quantity of non-protein-bound CO_2 (measured with serum electrolytes, in mEq/L)
ΔCO_2	=	Delta CO_2; difference between normal serum CO_2 and measured serum CO_2
COHb	=	Carboxyhemoglobin, usually expressed as a percentage of the total hemoglobin (e.g., 10% COHb)
CvO_2	=	Mixed venous oxygen content
dL	=	Deciliter, equals 100 mL
DPG	=	Diphosphoglycerate
Fe	=	Iron
FEV-1	=	Forced expiratory volume in the first second
FIO_2	=	Fraction of inspired oxygen, expressed either as a decimal (0.21, 1.00) or as a percent (21%, 100%)
FVC	=	Forced vital capacity
g	=	Gram
h	=	hours

$[H^+]$ = Hydrogen ion concentration, in nmoL/L
Hb = Hemoglobin
HCl = Hydrochloric acid
HCO_3^- = Bicarbonate
H–H = Henderson–Hasselbalch
K^+ = Potassium ion
L = liter, equals 1000 mL
mEq/L = milliequivalents/liter
MetHb = Methemoglobin
mg = Milligram
min = Minute
mL = Milliliter
mm Hg = Millimeters of mercury; standard unit for pressure, some texts use the term *torr;* 1 torr = 1 mm Hg
N_2 = Nitrogen
Na^+ = Sodium ion
O_2 = Oxygen
P or p = Pressure
P_{50} = PaO_2 at which 50% of the hemoglobin binding sites are combined with oxygen
$P(A–a)O_2$ = Difference between calculated alveolar PO_2 and measured arterial PO_2
P_B = Barometric pressure
$PetCO_2$ = Partial pressure of CO_2 measured on an end-tidal sample of expired air
pH = Negative logarithm of the hydrogen ion concentration, in nanomoles/liter
P_{H_2O} = Water vapor pressure
PIO_2 = Pressure of inspired oxygen
pK = Negative logarithm of the dissociation constant for carbonic acid (equals 6.1)
PvO_2 = Mixed venous partial pressure of oxygen
QT = Cardiac output
R or RQ = Respiratory quotient
SaO_2 = Saturation of hemoglobin with oxygen in arterial blood
SpO_2 = Saturation of hemoglobin with oxygen in arterial blood when measured with a pulse oximeter
torr = Unit of pressure; 1 torr = 1 mm Hg
V = Volume (e.g., VD = volume of dead space), in mL or L

$\dot{V}$	=	Volume per unit of time (e.g., see $\dot{V}O_2$)
VA	=	Alveolar volume, in mL or L
$\dot{V}A$	=	Alveolar ventilation, in L/min
VD	=	Dead space volume, in mL or L
$\dot{V}D$	=	Dead space ventilation, in L/min
$\dot{V}E$	=	Minute ventilation (usually measured on an expired sample, hence the *E*), in L/min
$\dot{V}O_2$	=	Oxygen uptake by the tissues, in mL/min
V–Q	=	Ventilation–perfusion; some texts place a dot above each letter, omitted here
VT	=	tidal volume, mL or L

APPENDIX

D

Glossary

Acetazolamide. A carbonic anhydrase inhibitor that prevents reabsorption of HCO_3^- in the renal tubule. Used as a drug in some cases of metabolic alkalosis to lower serum HCO_3^-; also used to prevent high-altitude sickness.

Acidemia. Acid in blood; indicates arterial pH < 7.35.

Acidosis. A physiologic process that, occurring alone, leads to an acidemia. Clinical causes include low-perfusion lactic acidosis (metabolic acidosis) and hypoventilation (respiratory acidosis).

Air. The mixture of gases that makes up the Earth's atmosphere; contains 78% nitrogen, 21% oxygen, 1% other gases.

Alkalemia. Alkali in blood; indicates arterial pH > 7.45.

Alkalosis. A physiologic process that, occurring alone, leads to an alkalemia. Causes include diuretic therapy (metabolic alkalosis) and acute hyperventilation (respiratory alkalosis).

Alveolar gas equation. Calculates PAO_2, the mean alveolar PO_2: $PAO_2 = PIO_2 - 1.2(PaCO_2)$.

Alveolar ventilation ($\dot{V}A$). The volume of air per minute that enters the alveoli and takes part in gas exchange; equals the total (minute) ventilation minus the dead space ventilation.

Alveolar–arterial PO_2 difference [$P(A\text{–}a)O_2$]. Difference between the calculated mean alveolar PO_2 and the measured arterial PO_2; colloquially called the *A–a gradient*. Elevation usually signifies a ventilation–perfusion imbalance within the lungs.

Anion gap. The difference between the serum sodium and the sum of chloride and bicarbonate concentrations; the normal AG is 12 ± 4 mEq/L. Elevation signifies excess unmeasured anions and a state of metabolic acidosis.

Atmosphere. The gaseous covering the surface of the Earth; approximately 150 miles in depth. Beyond the atmosphere is outer space.

Barometric pressure (P_B). Pressure of the atmosphere at a given altitude. At sea level, the pressure is 760 mm Hg, i.e., it will support a closed column of mercury 760 mm high.

Base excess. Difference between the normal quantity of total buffer base ([BB]) and the [BB] calculated from a blood sample; the normal BE is 0 ± 2 mEq/L. Elevation correlates with an increase in serum bicarbonate; reduction (negative BE) correlates with reduced bicarbonate.

Bicarbonate gap. Difference between the change in the anion gap and the change in serum CO_2; a definitely abnormal bicarbonate gap (outside range of ± 6 mEq/L) in the presence of an increased anion gap indicates some type of mixed acid–base disorder.

Bicarbonate (HCO_3^-). One of two buffer components of the bicarbonate buffering system; the normal HCO_3^- is 22-26 mEq/L.

Blood gas. Any gas dissolved in the blood, e.g., oxygen, nitrogen, carbon dioxide, or carbon monoxide; also refers to the test that measures partial pressure of oxygen (PO_2) and carbon dioxide (PCO_2), and pH.

Bronchitis. Inflammation of the airways; may be acute or chronic. Chronic bronchitis is often associated with cigarette smoking and may lead to chronic obstructive pulmonary disease.

Carbon dioxide (CO_2). A gaseous by-product of animal metabolism and the major determinant of acidity of the blood. Its partial pressure is routinely measured as part of arterial blood gases.

Carbon monoxide (CO). Colorless, odorless gas that combines avidly with hemoglobin to form carboxyhemoglobin; small amounts of inhaled CO can cause profound hypoxemia. Symptoms of CO poisoning usually begin when the level of carboxyhemoglobin exceeds 10%.

Carboxyhemoglobin. Hemoglobin bound with carbon monoxide.

Chronic obstructive pulmonary disease (COPD). Disease manifested by obstruction of the larger airways (> 2 mm in diameter) that does not normalize despite optimal therapy. Can be divided into two broad conditions, chronic bronchitis and emphysema, both of which are usually caused by long-term cigarette smoking.

Compensation. Alteration of the HCO_3^- or $PaCO_2$ in direct response to a primary acid–base disturbance, e.g., hyperventilation as a compensation for metabolic acidosis.

Confidence band. Area on an acid–base map that includes 95% of the compensatory responses of a group of subjects to one of the four primary acid–base disorders.

Co-oximeter. Machine capable of measuring SaO_2, carboxyhemoglobin, methemoglobin, and hemoglobin content from a single blood sample, using four wavelengths of light. Used in blood gas labs in addition to the blood gas analyzer, which measures PO_2, PCO_2, and pH.

Cyanosis. Blue color of skin and mucous membranes, usually apparent when the desaturated (reduced) hemoglobin content in the capillaries exceeds 5 g/dL.

Dead space ventilation. The volume of air per minute that enters the airways (including the alveoli) and does not take part in gas exchange; the volume of air that enters the physiologic dead space each minute. Dead space ventilation equals total (minute) ventilation minus alveolar ventilation.

Dead space. Space that contains air but doesn't allow for gas exchange. *Anatomic* dead space is made up of all nonalveolar air spaces (upper airway and all bronchi, including terminal bronchioles). *Physiologic* dead space includes all the anatomic dead space plus the alveolar spaces that don't take part in gas exchange. Anatomic dead space is fixed in a given patient; physiologic dead space varies according to the extent and severity of the ventilation–perfusion imbalance.

Denitrogenation. Process of removing nitrogen from the blood by inhaling 100% oxygen.

Diffusion. Physiologic process by which respiratory gases are exchanged across cell membranes; all diffusion in the respiratory system takes place from a region of higher gas pressure across a permeable membrane to a region of lower gas pressure.

Electrolytes. Positively or negatively charged ions in the blood; the most commonly measured electrolytes are sodium (Na^+), potassium (K^+), bicarbonate (HCO_3^-), and chloride (Cl^-).

Emphysema. One type of chronic obstructive pulmonary disease; manifested by destruction of the alveolar–capillary membranes and an increased ventilation–perfusion imbalance.

End-capillary. In the pulmonary circulation, the last section of capillary that exchanges gases with the alveoli; in normal lungs, the end-capillary PO_2 and PCO_2 of an individual gas exchange unit are assumed to equal the corresponding alveolar PO_2 and PCO_2, respectively.

End-tidal. The last portion of exhaled tidal volume; in normal lungs the end-tidal PCO_2 is assumed equal to the alveolar PCO_2, because alveolar gas is the last portion to leave the lungs during exhalation.

Ferric iron (Fe^{+++}). Iron in the oxidized state; heme groups that contain ferric iron cannot bind oxygen.

Ferrous iron (Fe^{++}). Iron in its normal state combined with hemoglobin.

Flow. Volume per unit time, measured, for example, in L/min or L/s.

Forced expiratory volume in the first second (FEV-1). That portion of the forced vital capacity exhaled in the first second of effort.

Forced vital capacity (FVC). Volume of air that can be rapidly and forcibly exhaled after a maximal inhalation.

Gas. Any matter that will expand in three dimensions to fill the available space.

Helium. A lightweight, inert gas; used to measure lung volumes in the helium–dilution lung function test.

Heme. Iron–porphyrin portion of the hemoglobin that chemically binds with oxygen.

Hemoglobin. Iron–porphyrin–protein complex that chemically binds oxygen, thus allowing for much greater oxygen–carrying capacity than can be achieved from dissolved oxygen alone. Each molecule of hemoglobin is capable of combining with four molecules of oxygen.

Henderson–Hasselbalch equation. Relates pH to the HCO_3^-:$PaCO_2$ ratio.

Hypercapnia. Elevated $PaCO_2$ ($>$ 45 mm Hg).

Hypercarbia. Elevated HCO_3^- (plasma $HCO_3^- > 26$ mEq/L).

Hyperventilation. Excessive alveolar ventilation for the amount of CO_2 production; hyperventilation results in a fall in $PaCO_2$.

Hypocapnia. Reduced $PaCO_2$ (< 35 mm Hg).

Hypocarbia. Reduced HCO_3^- ($HCO_3^- < 22$ mEq/L)

Hypoventilation. Alveolar ventilation decreased for the amount of CO_2 production; hypoventilation results in a rise in $PaCO_2$.

Hypoxemia. Reduced PaO_2 and/or arterial oxygen content ($PaO_2 < 60$ mm Hg or $SaO_2 < 90\%$).

Hypoxia. General reduction in oxygen delivery, either because of hypoxemia, decreased cardiac output, or decreased oxygen uptake in the systemic capillaries.

Inert gas. A gas that does not enter into any chemical reaction with another substance; examples include hydrogen, helium, nitrogen, and argon.

Metabolic acidosis. A primary physiologic process that, occurring alone, causes acidemia by lowering the HCO_3^-. Causes include low-perfusion lactic acidosis, keto-acidosis, and aspirin overdose.

Metabolic alkalosis. A primary physiologic process that, occurring alone, causes alkalemia by raising the HCO_3^-. Causes include diuretic therapy, corticosteroids, and nasogastric suction.

Methemoglobin. Hemoglobin that contains iron in its oxidized state (Fe^{+++}); in this state, hemoglobin cannot bind oxygen.

Minute ventilation ($\dot{V}E$). Same as total ventilation; the amount of air inhaled or exhaled per minute. By convention, minute ventilation is measured on exhalation.

Mixed venous blood. Blood in the pulmonary artery, i.e., blood that is a mixture of the total venous return to the right side of the heart.

Nanomole. One-billionth of a mole; hydrogen ions are quantified in nanomoles, e.g., a pH of 7.40 represents a $[H^+]$ of 40 nmol/L.

Nitrogen. Inert gas that makes up 78% of air.

Obstructive impairment. Caused by decreased air flow through the bronchi; usually manifested by reduction in the FEV-1:FVC ratio.

Oxidized hemoglobin. Hemoglobin that contains iron in its oxidized state (Fe^{+++}); synonymous with methemoglobin.

Oximetry. Noninvasive method of measuring arterial oxygen saturation;

modern machines measure pulse at the same time, hence the test is sometimes referred to as pulse oximetry.

Oxygen content. The quantity of oxygen in the blood (in mL O_2/dL).

Oxygen dissociation curve. Sigmoid curve obtained when values for SaO_2 are plotted in relation to the corresponding PaO_2 values. Shifts of the O_2 dissociation curve to the right or to the left can affect oxygen delivery to the tissues.

Oxygen saturation. The percentage of total hemoglobin binding sites chemically combined with oxygen; the maximum is 100%. The normal oxygen saturation is 95–98%.

Oxygen. Respirable gas essential to life; oxygen makes up 21% of the atmosphere.

Partial pressure. Pressure exerted by a single gas; partial pressure is unaffected by any other gases that may be present. The sum of all partial pressures equals the total gas pressure, which in air is the same as barometric pressure.

Peak flow. Maximal flow rate attained on forced exhalation after maximal inhalation (in L/min or L/s).

Perfusion. Amount of blood circulating to an area or organ per minute.

Physiologic dead space. Volume of all airways, including alveoli, that contain air but do not participate in gas exchange.

Pressure. Force exerted by molecules; gas pressure is determined by the number and speed of molecules that make up the gas. All gases exert pressure when free and uncombined chemically with a non-gas molecule. When oxygen or carbon dioxide chemically combine with hemoglobin, they no longer exert any pressure.

Pulse oximeter. Machine that sends two wavelengths of light through a digit (or ear lobe) and noninvasively measure hemoglobin oxygen saturation; compare with co-oximeter.

Reduced hemoglobin. Hemoglobin that is not combined with oxygen; contains iron in its normal, ferrous state (Fe^{++}).

Respiratory acidosis. Acid–base state manifested by elevated $PaCO_2$ and reduced pH.

Respiratory alkalosis. Acid–base state manifested by reduced $PaCO_2$ and elevated pH.

Respiratory failure. Any state manifested by a low PaO_2 and/or high $PaCO_2$ that is caused by a defect in the respiratory system. Indicates $PaO_2 <$ 60 mm Hg or $PaCO_2 >$ 50 mm Hg while breathing room air at sea level; different criteria apply for other conditions.

Restrictive impairment. Respiratory impairment manifested by an inability to inhale maximally and, therefore a decreased total lung capacity. Caused by many conditions, both within and outside the lungs, e.g., pleural effusion, pulmonary fibrosis, congestive heart failure, neuromuscular weakness, and obesity.

Shunt. Blood flowing through the lungs that does not come into contact with air; may be from anatomic causes (e.g., an arteriovenous fistula) or physiologic causes. A physiologic shunt occurs when alveoli become unventilated (e.g., from atelectasis) but remain perfused (V-Q = zero for those units).

Spirometry. Breathing test that measures vital capacity and its subdivisions.

Supplemental oxygen. Oxygen delivered to a patient at a greater percentage than in the atmosphere; $FIO_2 > 21\%$.

Tidal volume. Volume of air inhaled or exhaled during a normal quiet breath.

Torr. Unit of pressure; 1 torr = 1 mm Hg.

Ventilation. Amount of air entering the lungs per minute; the total or minute ventilation is the sum of the dead space and alveolar ventilation.

Ventilation–perfusion (ventilation/perfusion). The ratio of ventilation to perfusion in a single alveolus, a region of the lungs, or both lungs.

Ventilation–perfusion imbalance. When there is more, or less, than the normal amount of ventilation for the amount of perfusion to an alveolus or a group of alveoli. V–Q imbalance is the main physiologic cause of a decrease in PaO_2. Occurs when some lung units are relatively underventilated or relatively overperfused; many lung diseases lead to a ventilation–perfusion imbalance.

APPENDIX

E

References

Preface

Clark LC Jr. Monitoring and control of blood and tissue O_2 tensions. Trans Am Soc Artif Intern Organs 1956;2:41.

Clark LC Jr, Wolf R, Granger D, Taylor Z. Continuous recording of blood oxygen tensions by polarography. J Appl Physiol 1953;6:189.

Comroe JH Jr. Physiology of respiration. 2nd ed. Chicago: Mosby-Year Book, 1974.

Severinghaus JW. AHA! Chapter XVIII in Astrup P, Severinghaus JW. The history of blood gases, acids and bases. Copenhagen: Radiometer A/S, Copenhagen 1986.

Stadie WC. The oxygen of the arterial and venous blood in pneumonia and its relation to cyanosis. J Exp Med 1919;30:215.

Chapter 3

Callaham M, Barton C. Prediction of outcome of cardiopulmonary resuscitation from end-tidal carbon dioxide concentration. Crit Care Med 1990;18:358.

Clark JS, Votteri B, Ariagno R, et al. Noninvasive assessment of blood gases: state of the art. Am Rev Respir Dis 1992;145:220.

Eriksson L, Wollmer P, Olsson CG, et al. Diagnosis of pulmonary embolism based upon alveolar dead space analysis. Chest 1989;96:357.

Hatle L, Rokseth R. The arterial to end-expiratory carbon dioxide tension gradient in acute pulmonary embolism and other cardiopulmonary diseases. Chest 1974;66:352.

Isserles S, Breen PH. Can changes in end-tidal PCO_2 measure changes in cardiac output? Anesth Analg 1991;73:808.

Levine RL, Wayne MA, Miller CC. End-tidal carbon dioxide and outcome of out-of-hospital cardiac arrest. New Engl J Med 1997;337:301.

Liu SY, Lee TS, Bongard F. Accuracy of capnography in nonintubated surgical patients. Chest 1992;102:1512.

Moorthy SS, Losasso AM, Wilcox J. End-tidal PCO_2 greater than $PaCO_2$. Chest 1984;12:534.

Sanders AB, Kern KB, Otto CW, et al. End-tidal carbon dioxide monitoring during cardiopulmonary resuscitation: a prognostic indicator for survival. JAMA 1989;262:1347.

Shibutani K, Muraoka M, Shirasaki S. Do changes in end-tidal PCO_2 quantitatively reflect changes in cardiac output? Anesth Analg 1994;79:829.

Shibutani K, Shirasaki S, Braaz T, et al. Changes in cardiac output affect $PETco_2$, CO_2 transport, and O_2 uptake during unsteady state in humans. J Clin Monit 1992;8:175–176.

Stock MC. Capnography for adults. Crit Care Clinics 1995;11:219.

Wright SW. Conscious sedation in the emergency department: the value of capnography and pulse oximetry. Ann Emerg Med 1992;21:93.

Chapter 4

Cinel D, Markwell K, Lee R, Szidon P. Variability of the respiratory gas exchange ratio during arterial puncture. Am Rev Respir Dis 1991;143:217.

Gowda M, Klocke RA. Variability of indices of hypoxemia in adult respiratory distress syndrome. Crit Care Med 1997;25:41. See also Letters. Crit Care Med 1997;25:1612, 1437.

Martin L. Abbreviating the alveolar gas equation. An argument for simplicity. Respir Care 1986;31:40.

Sorbini CA, Grassi V, Solinas E, Muiesan G. Arterial oxygen tension in relation to age in healthy subjects. Respiration 1968;25:3.

West JB, Hackett PH, Maret KH, et al. Pulmonary gas exchange on the summit of Mt. Everest, J Appl Physiol 1983;55:678.

Chapter 5

Comroe JH Jr, Botelho S. The unreliability of cyanosis in the recognition of arterial hypoxemia. Am J Med Sci 1947;214:1.

Lundsgaard C, Van Slyke DD. Cyanosis. Medicine 1923;2:1.

Martin L, Khalil H. How much reduced hemoglobin is necessary to generate central cyanosis? Chest 1990;97:182.

Chapter 6

Ayas N, Bergstrom LR, Schwab TR, et al. Unrecognized severe postoperative hypercapnia: a case of apneic oxygenation. Mayo Clin Proc 1998;73:51.

Barker SJ, Tremper KK. The effect of carbon monoxide inhalation on pulse oximetry and transcutaneous PO_2. Anesthesiology 1987;66:677.

Barker SJ, Tremper KK, Hyatt J. Effects of methemoglobinemia on pulse oximetry and mixed venous oximetry. Anesthesiology 1989;70:112.

Clark JS, Votteri B, Ariagno R, et al. Noninvasive assessment of blood gases: state of the art. Am Rev Respir Dis 1992;145:220.

Coté CJ, Goldstein A, Fuchsman WH, et al. The effect of nail polish on pulse oximetry. Anesth Analg 1988;67:683.

Council on Scientific Affairs, American Medical Association. The use of pulse oximetry during conscious sedation. JAMA 1993;270:1463.

Davidson JAH, Hosie HE. Limitations of pulse oximetry: respiratory insufficiency—a failure of detection. Brit Med J 1993;307:372.

Eisenkraft JB. Pulse oximeter desaturation due to methemoglobinemia. Anesthesiology 1988;68:279.

Ernst A, Zibrak JD. Carbon monoxide poisoning. New Engl J Med 1998; 339:1603–1608.

Hampson NB. Pulse oximetry in severe carbon monoxide poisoning. Chest 1998;144:1036–1041.

Hanning CD, Alexander-Williams JM. Pulse oximetry: a practical review. Brit Med J 1995;311:367.

Hutton P, Clutton-Brock T. The benefits and pitfalls of pulse oximetry. Brit Med J 1993;307:457.

Leasa DJ, Technology Subcommittee of the Working Group on Critical Care. Noninvasive blood gas monitoring: a review of the use in the adult critical care unit. Can Med Assoc J 1992;146:703.

Lindberg LG, Lennmarken C, Vegfors M. Pulse oximetry—clinical implications and recent technical developments. Acta Anaesth Scand 1995;39:279.

Raemer DN, Elliott WR, Topulos G, et al. The theoretical effect of carboxyhemoglobin on the pulse oximeter. J Clin Monit 1989;5:246.

Ralston AC, Webb RK, Runciman WB. Potential errors in pulse oximetry. III: Effects of interference, dyes, dyshaemoglobins and other pigments. Anaesthesia 1991;46:291.

Ries AL, Prewitt LM, Johnson JJ. Skin color and ear oximetry. Chest 1989;96:287.

Schnapp LM, Cohen NH. Pulse oximetry: uses and abuses. Chest 1990; 98:1244.

Severinghaus JW, Astrup PB. History of blood gas analysis. VI. Oximetry. J Clin Monit 1986;2:270–188.

Severinghaus JW, Kelleher JF. Recent developments in pulse oximetry. Anesthesiology 1992;76:1018.

Stoneham MD, Saville GM, Wilson IH. Knowledge about pulse oximetry among medical and nursing staff. Lancet 1994;344:1339.

Veyckemans F, Baele P, Guillaume JE, et al. Hyperbilirubinemia does not interfere with hemoglobin saturation measured by pulse oximetry. Anesthesiology 1989;70:118.

Wahr JA, Tremper KK. Noninvasive oxygen monitoring techniques. Crit Care Clin 1995;11:199.

Watcha MF, Connor MT, Hing AV. Pulse oximetry in met-hemoglobinemia. Am J Dis Child 1989;143:845.

Zeballos RJ, Weisman IM. Reliability of noninvasive oximetry in black subjects during exercise and hypoxia. Am Rev Resp Dis 1991;144:1240.

Chapter 7

Campbell EJM. RipH. Lancet 1962;1:681.

Emmett M, Narins RG. Clinical use of the anion gap. Medicine (Baltimore) 1977;56:38.

Gabow PA, principal discussant. Disorders associated with an altered anion gap. Kidney Int 1985;27:472.

Gabow PA, Kaehny WD, Fennessy PV, et al. Diagnostic importance of an increased serum anion gap. N Engl J Med 1980; 303:854.

Haber RJ. A practical approach to acid-base disorders. West J Med 1991;155:146.

Hills AG. pH and the Henderson-Hasselbalch equation. Am J Med 1973;55:131.

Hood I, Campbell EJM. Is pK OK? (Editorial) N Engl J Med 1982;306:864.

Lennon EJ, Lemann J Jr. pH—is it defensible? Ann Intern Med 1966;65:1151.

Narins RG, Emmett M. Simple and mixed acid-base disorders: a practical approach. Medicine (Baltimore) 1980;59:161.

Oh MS, Carroll HJ. The anion gap. N Engl J Med 1977;297:814.

Oster JR, Perez GO, Materson BJ. Use of the anion gap in clinical medicine. South Med J 1988;81:229.

Paulson WD, Gadallah MF. Diagnosis of mixed acid-base disorders in diabetic ketoacidosis. Am J Med Sci 1993;306:295.

Sadjadi SA. A new range for the anion gap. Ann Intern Med 1995;123:807.

Winter SD, Pearson JR, Gabow PA, et al. The fall of the serum anion gap. Arch Intern Med 1990;150:311.

Wrenn K. The delta (Δ) gap: an approach to mixed acid-base disorders. Ann Emerg Med 1990;19:1310.

Chapter 8

Arbus GS, Hebert LA, Levesque PR, et al. Characterization and clinical application of the "significance band" for acute respiratory alkalosis. N Engl J Med 1969;280:117.

Asch MJ, Dell RB, Williams GS, et al. Time course for development of respiratory compensation in metabolic acidosis. J Lab Clin Med 1969;73:610.

Brackett NC Jr, Cohen JJ, Schwartz WB. Carbon dioxide titration curve of normal man. N Engl J Med 1965;272:6.

Javaheri S. Compensatory hypoventilation in metabolic alkalosis. Chest 1982;81:296.

Javaheri S, Kazemi H. Metabolic alkalosis and hypoventilation in humans. Am Rev Respir Dis 1987:136;1011.

Narins RG, Emmett M. Simple and mixed acid-base disorders: a practical approach. Medicine (Baltimore) 1980;59:161.

Pierce NF, Fedson DS, Brigham KL, et al. The ventilatory response to acute acid-base deficit in humans. Ann Intern Med 1970;72:633.

Winters RW. Terminology of acid-base disorders. Ann Intern Med 1965;63:873.

Chapter 12

Martin L. Pulmonary physiology in clinical practice. St. Louis: Mosby-Year Book, 1987.

Weil MH, Rackow EC, Trevino R, et al. Difference in acid-base state between venous and arterial blood during cardiopulmonary resuscitation. N Engl J Med 1986;315:153.

Chapter 13

Sacchetti A, Grynn J, Pope A, Vasso S. Leukocyte larceny: spurious hypoxemia confirmed with pulse oximetry. J Emerg Med 1990;8:567.

Suggested Reading

Journal Articles

Androgue HJ, Madias NE. Management of life-threatening acid-base disorders. New Engl J Med 1998;338:26, 107.

Clark LC Jr. Measurement of oxygen tension: a historical perspective. Crit Care Med 1981;9:690.

Hsia CCW. Respiratory function of hemoglobin. New Engl J Med 1998;338:239.

Mizock BA. Utility of standard base excess in acid-base analysis. Crit Care Med 1998;26:1146–1147.

Pilon CS, Leathley M, London R, et al. Practice guidelines for arterial blood gas measurement in the intensive care unit decreases numbers and increases appropriateness of tests. Crit Care Med 1997;25:1308.

Schwartz WB, Relman AS. A critique of the parameters used in evaluation of acid-base disorders. N Engl J Med 1963;268:1382.

Schlichtig R, Grogono AW, Severinghaus JW. Human $PaCO_2$ compensation and standard base excess compensation for acid-base imbalance. Crit Care Med 1998;26:1173–1179.

Severinghaus JW, Astrup P. History of blood gas analysis. Int Anesth Clin 1987;25:1–224.

Severinghaus JW, Astrup P, Murray JF. Blood gas analysis and critical care medicine. Am J Resp Crit Care Med 1998;157:S114.

Statement on acid-base terminology. Report of the ad hoc committee of the New York Academy of Sciences Conference, November 23–24, 1964. Ann Intern Med 1965;63:885.

Wahr JA, Tremper KK. Noninvasive oxygen monitoring techniques. Crit Care Clin 1995;11:199.

West JB. State of the art. Ventilation-perfusion relationships. Am Rev Respir Dis 1977;116:919.

Zimmerman JL, Dellinger RP. Blood gas monitoring. Crit Care Clinics 1996;12:865.

Books

Astrup P, Severinghaus JW. The history of blood gases, acids and bases. Copenhagen: Radiometer A/S, 1986.

Berne RM, Levy MN. Physiology. 4th ed. St. Louis: Mosby-Year Book, 1998.

Ganong WF. Review of medial physiology. Norwalk, CN: Appleton & Lange, 1995.

Guyton AC, Hall JE. Textbook of medical physiology. 9th ed. Philadelphia: Saunders, 1996.

Kokko JP, Tannen RL, eds. Fluids and electrolytes. 3rd ed. Philadelphia: Saunders, 1996.

Malley WJ. Clinical blood gases. application and non-invasive alternatives. Philadelphia: Saunders, 1990.

Prange HD. Respiratory physiology: understanding gas exchange. New York: Chapman & Hall, 1995.

Rose, BD. Clinical physiology of acid-base and electrolytes. 4th ed. New York: McGraw Hill, 1994.

Shapiro BA, Peruzzi WT, Kozelowski-Templin RL. Clinical application of blood gases. 5th ed. Chicago: Mosby-Year Book, 1994.

Tisi GM. Pulmonary physiology in clinical medicine. 3rd ed. Baltimore, MD: Williams & Wilkins, 1992.

West JB. Respiratory physiology—the essentials. 5th ed. Baltimore, MD: Williams & Wilkins, 1998.

West JB. Ventilation/blood flow and gas exchange. 5th ed. Philadelphia: Lippincott, 1990.

Index

Page numbers in *italics* denote figures; those followed by a t denote tables.